PAINTING TWO

A. Cloud of gray, magenta, and purple indicates that this person is viewing the world with sadness, individuality and creativity, and intuition.

B. Yellow head, antenna, and upper body indicates intuition, generosity, a spiritual teacher, and inner joy. The antennae indicate a search for creativity, authenticity, and intuition.

C. Large third eye.

D. Red dots indicate some anxiety.

E. Magenta in the 5th chakra reflects the need to express themselves authentically.

F. Arms raised in surrender to a new start. Orange for courage and adventurousness.

G, H. Blue means empathetic and sensitive. In this case, sensing other people's energy.

I. Purple in the gut indicates a need to trust the gut instincts.

J. Red dots in the 1st and 2nd chakras indicate early trauma.

K. The release of courage by addressing the trauma.

L. The release of the trauma.

M. Legs are about moving forward in life. Orange is acknowledging the courage needed to do so.

N. Magenta in the legs means that authenticity is needed in order to move forward.

O. Green is about growth and new life. Grounding will help facilitate that.

"YOU are capable of being your own medical intuitive, and Katie Beecher's book *Heal from Within* is just the sort of step-by-step guide you need. With clear instructions on how to open your own intuition, and identify the energy centers to focus on, she provides a roadmap for you to unblock your chakras and walk into your whole, healthy self. **If you're ready to take your physical, emotional, and spiritual health into your own hands and start to heal, this is the book you've been waiting for!**"

—Dana Childs, intuitive, energy healer, speaker, and coauthor of *Chakras, Food & You: Tap Your Individual Energy System for Health, Healing, and Harmonious Weight*

"It has been a long time since a self-help book grabbed me in this way. Katie Beecher has a gift for understanding the body and mind. Her intuitive gifts and teachings provide you with a real behind the scenes look at the way your energy system can impact all areas of your life. If you or a loved one are struggling with a chronic condition **this book will give you hope, inspiration and healing.**"

—Sherianna Boyle, author of *Emotional Detox Now*

"In this essential book, Katie Beecher combines her gifts in psychology and medical intuition to offer us a course in healing ourselves from the inside out. She teaches us practical steps for identifying the root causes of chronic conditions—physical, emotional, mental, and spiritual—and how to address them. This is a book to return to again and again."

—Cynthia Li, MD, integrative physician, and bestselling author of *Brave New Medicine*

"Holistic healing at it's best. This self-help manual gives you the opportunity to find out your true life purpose, become a spiritual intuitive, or enhance your practitioner skills for your own clients. Katie highlights her unique intuitive reading process using case studies, art, and chakras, and gives clues on how to harmonize these with guidance on the most appropriate modalities and nutritional support that will assist the healing process."

—Tim Fraser, former president of the Australian
Holistic Healers and Counsellors Association,
founder of Australian Doctor Healer Network

"*Heal from Within* is the perfect blend of physical, emotional, and spiritual information. Katie gives patients the knowledge and tools to take charge of their health, facilitating healing on all levels. A valuable resource for anyone struggling with health issues."

—Jessica Sedita, ND, naturopathic physician

"*Heal from Within* offers incredibly valuable insights on healing our most important relationship, the one we have with ourselves. Using a step-by-step, systematic approach, Katie takes us through the process of accessing our inner wisdom to find answers to both our emotional and physical ailments and how to heal them. Her wisdom and expertise as both a counselor and a medical intuitive makes this a valuable resource you will turn to time and time again. It's not often a book on healing addresses the complex dimensions of mind, body, and spirit so thoroughly and yet so understandably. Her clarity can help you achieve your own and that is a special gift."

—Kris Ferraro, healer, coach, and Amazon bestselling
author of *Energy Healing* and *Manifesting*

HEAL
FROM
WITHIN

HEAL
FROM
WITHIN

A Guidebook to
Intuitive Wellness

KATIE BEECHER, MS, LPC

ST. MARTIN'S
ESSENTIALS
NEW YORK

First published in the United States by St. Martin's Essentials, an imprint of St. Martin's Publishing Group

www.stmartins.com

Library of Congress Cataloging-in-Publication Data

Names: Beecher, Katie, author.
Title: Heal from within : a guidebook to intuitive wellness / Katie Beecher, MS, LPC.
Description: First Edition. | New York, NY : St. Martin's Essentials, [2022] | Includes bibliographical references and index.
Identifiers: LCCN 2021047612 | ISBN 9781250780249 (hardcover) | ISBN 9781250780256 (ebook)
Subjects: LCSH: Self-actualization (Psychology) | Mind and body. | Spirituality.
Classification: LCC BF637.S4 B4254 2022 | DDC 158—dc23
LC record available at https://lccn.loc.gov/2021047612

Our books may be purchased in bulk for promotional, educational, or business use. Please contact your local bookseller or the Macmillan Corporate and Premium Sales Department at 1-800-221-7945, extension 5442, or by email at MacmillanSpecialMarkets@macmillan.com.

First Edition: 2022

10 9 8 7 6 5 4 3 2 1

To my husband Brad and daughters Lauren and Larissa, who have been my inspiration and unwavering supporters. I am beyond grateful to get to share my life with them.

CONTENTS

Introduction   1

PART I

1. How to Use This Book   7

2. What I Believe   13

3. Finding My Life Purpose   19

4. My Unique, Individual Reading Process   27

5. You Are Never Alone: Connecting to Intuition   37

6. Symptoms Are Signals from Our Intuition   55

7. Identifying Individual Issues and Strengths   59

8. The Complete Person: Healing Using the 7th Chakra   82

9. Intuitive Sight, Wisdom, and Truth: Healing Using
the 6th Chakra   92

10. Finding Your Voice: Healing Using the 5th Chakra   112

11. "Don't Be So Sensitive": Healing Using the
4th Chakra   129

12. Self-Esteem, Body Image, and the Gut-Brain:
    Healing Using the 3rd Chakra   140

13. Sex, Power, and Life Purpose: Healing Using the
    2nd Chakra   159

14. Trust, Safety, Security, and Family: Healing Using
    the 1st Chakra   175

PART II

Glossary of Healing   195

Epilogue: How to Use This Book Going Forward   269

Acknowledgments: With Love and Gratitude   271

Appendix: Websites, Resources, Healing Therapies,
and Recommended Products   273

Notes   279

Index   281

Chakra Chart Worksheet   291

Introduction

Through pride we are ever deceiving ourselves. But deep
down below the surface of the average conscience a still,
small voice says to us, something is out of tune.

—Carl Jung

*With connection to intuition, self-love, and acceptance, we can
heal from anything.* This is the message I received from my intuitive guides at the age of sixteen, when they told me I would
be writing this book as a result of what I had learned while
recovering from bulimia. I have never forgotten it.

Some of the most serious, painful, chronic, and difficult to
heal "illnesses" I have experienced and witnessed have been
sparked by incredibly challenging life circumstances. At the
same time, some of the most profound healing and growth I
have experienced, and have watched clients experience, has
come as a by-product of similarly difficult and painful experiences. When we are struggling with illness, it is essential to
identify and address not only physical root issues but also everything in our past and present that may be contributing to
being "unwell," whether that be physically, emotionally, and/or
spiritually. We must also identify everything that can contribute to healing. Trauma, our relationships and careers, what we
put into and on our bodies, family influences, our relationship
with Spirit and/or God, creativity, our empathic and intuitive

abilities, and our ability to be authentic and heard can all have an impact on our wellness.

This is what my work and *Heal from Within* are all about.

I know that what I have just said is true because all of my personal healing and growth, all of the self-discovery, even my work as a medical intuitive has been the result of honestly identifying and addressing the issues that were blocking me from reaching my full potential. I also know this is true because I have had the pleasure of helping thousands of people do the same.

I'm not going to pretend it is easy. Healing this way can be hard and a lot of work. It will also be the most rewarding thing you have ever done for yourself. The most difficult thing I have ever done was recover from bulimia, because I had to learn to love myself. Over the past thirty years of recovery, my eating disorder has been my greatest gift because it permanently changed my life for the better.

In order to heal, I had to learn to accept and address my fears of being seen and heard, of being imperfect, and of possibly never feeling worthy of love. I had to accept the fact that I couldn't and shouldn't be in control all the time and that a stronger, higher force had my back. I had to risk trusting others and myself and learn to ask for help.

I also had to face the fact that much of the pain I had been living with for so long had been created by my dysfunctional family, the people who were supposed to love me but were not capable of giving me what I needed. In order to grow, heal, and ultimately find my life path and voice, I had to call up courage and strength I didn't even realize I possessed. Unfortunately, my story is far from unique, and I hear similar stories on an almost daily basis. If you are willing to put in the work, you truly can put your pain behind you and embrace the life you have always wanted.

Heal from Within is the first book to combine information from personal spiritual guides with the wisdom of medical intuition, clinical counseling experience, and specific healing tools from Jungian psychology. You will be able to use it as a working guide both now and for years to come. The tools and concepts in *Heal from Within* are the same ones I have been imparting to my clients as a medical intuitive and counselor for the past thirty years, and I am thrilled to be teaching them to you.

You may be one of the millions of people living with one or more chronic conditions, which, according to the CDC website, six in ten Americans have, and four in ten have more than one. By 2030, it is predicted that two of every five individuals will be living with three or more chronic health conditions.

You don't have to continue to suffer. The path to your relief and health rejuvenation is at hand. You already have the ability and knowledge to help yourself; this book will teach you how to unlock it.

The answer is likely not to be found in traditional medicine or in the ways we are currently caring for our sick and hurting population. A report from the Commonwealth Fund found that even though the United States leads the world in healthcare spending, its residents are more ill and more likely to die of preventable conditions than those in similarly wealthy and developed countries. Many of the people who contact me are on the verge of giving up. They have worked with numerous traditional and alternative practitioners, often spending thousands of dollars, without making progress, without receiving answers, and often ending up feeling even worse.

The answer to your wellness crisis starts by communicating with your own intuition: a force within all of us that provides endless love, guidance, protection, and security. When we form a strong connection with our intuition, we can heal from anything. By enlisting our intuition to help discover and address the root causes of illness and unhappiness, and by using individualized strategies and remedies that fit our specific needs, lifestyle, genetics, and unique bodies, we can achieve true, lasting health and live the authentic lives we all strive to achieve.

How can I be so sure? I know this because I have personally watched people's lives transform physically, emotionally, and spiritually. I've seen clients go from being bedridden to walking four miles a day, from being engulfed by suicidal depression to leading a life of joy and productivity, from being told that an organ transplant was necessary to a seemingly impossible organ rejuvenation, and from being captive in abusive relationships to living with independence and incredible self-esteem. They used the very same techniques you are about to learn in *Heal from Within*.

PART I

How to Use This Book

Knowing your own darkness is the best method for dealing
with the darknesses of other people.

—Carl Jung

This book is a comprehensive plan for health and wellness that
you will want to refer to again and again, not just use one time
for a specific issue. The tools are timeless and are designed to
be adjusted to meet the needs of individuals of all ages as they
move through their lives.

Clients will often come to me looking for advice on supplements, nutrition, testing, or other physical types of relief,
without realizing that they have other work to do. That work
is sometimes dialing into the terrifying fear, shame, and self-
loathing that is preventing them from healing. If we do not
allow our intuition to be in charge and direct our healing,
permanent change isn't possible. The good news is that the
answers are already inside each one of us, just waiting to be
found.

This book will help you find those answers, beginning by
helping you identify the emotional, spiritual, and physical
root causes for your issues. These issues are unique to you
as an individual, which is why one-size-fits-all protocols and

testing often are not successful. I will teach you *my* definition of intuition and my special techniques for connection with it, which you can use to enhance all areas of your life. I will guide you toward assembling treatment and wellness plans to fit your lifestyle, individual needs, and dietary preferences, using detailed questionnaires, checklists, and of course your intuition, to help you, now and in the future. I will also help you choose other appropriate wellness and medical professionals to help you in your health journey, just as I do in my practice. Working with a team of experts assures that as many bases as possible are covered. I work with and recommend other practitioners on a regular basis who can verify the findings of my guides using their experience and various means of testing.

This book is not a substitute for medical advice and I am not a doctor. I am a licensed professional counselor, so I can give advice about mental health issues, but this book is not a substitute for individualized therapy. The information in this book comes from my intuitive guides, over thirty years of professional intuitive counseling experience, life experience, techniques from Jungian psychology, and recommendations from other health professionals. Whether in this book or in my practice, it is very important to me that the information I provide be scientifically sound and responsible. I do not have space here to give research citations for every recommendation, but I will provide them as much as possible, and I encourage you to do your own research.

This book is a program designed to be followed *step-by-step*, chapter-by-chapter. Traditional models of health and healing begin by focusing on one main problem or symptom, usually emotional or physical, treating the symptom, then waiting for the problem to reappear or progressing to the next problem or symptom. This method does not treat the whole person and doesn't work in the long term.

WE WILL BE DOING THINGS DIFFERENTLY!

I will teach you to connect to your intuition so you can begin using it to identify what you want to work on as well as your strengths. You will also use it to help make decisions regarding healing and wellness.

Next, you will identify your issues—emotional, physical, and spiritual—as well as the root causes, using the main energy centers in your body so you get a complete picture.

You will prioritize what you would like to tackle first and use your intuition and the detailed information provided to choose which healing strategies best fit your specific symptoms, lifestyle, and beliefs.

The investigative and healing chapters of the book (8 through 14) are arranged by chakras, the seven main energy centers of the body, each with corresponding parts of the body, along with emotional and spiritual characteristics. In each chapter, I offer advice about the general issues associated with each chakra, as well as information about certain specific conditions and diseases. The second part of the book contains a list of specific conditions you can reference, along with recommendations tailored to each.

I have organized the chapters in this book in the same way that I conduct my readings, since I know this process works, for every type of question and issue.

Chapter 1 gives you a road map of how to use this book, now and for many years to come.

The second chapter gives you an outline of my basic principles and beliefs. These are things I have come to learn over my thirty-plus years of practice and that I've learned from my intuitive guides.

Chapter 3 touches on the two subjects I'm most frequently

asked about: the start of my healing journey and how I discovered my medical intuitive abilities and life purpose. Over the course of my life, I learned to embrace my spiritual gifts instead of being terrified of them, and now I spend my life healing and teaching others.

The fourth chapter contains a description of how I conduct my individual medical and spiritual intuitive readings and explains how you too will be able to use a similar method for your own healing.

Chapter 5 will teach you techniques for connecting to your intuition and your body. This is one of the most important chapters in the book. Connection to intuition literally saved my life. You will use your intuition throughout the book to help identify your issues and their root causes and facilitate healing and lasting wellness.

Chapter 6 is about how your body and intuition use symptoms as symbols to communicate with you and get your attention.

In Chapter 7, you will identify your individual issues and strengths. This chapter contains descriptions of the seven major energetic healing centers of the body, or chakras, and tools for how to use them to identify your individual issues as well as some of the possible physical, emotional, and spiritual root causes. *Chakra* is a Sanskrit term for "wheels of energy and light," which originated approximately three thousand years ago in India. When our energy in or moving through these chakras is blocked or disturbed (much more about that later), we develop physical, emotional, and spiritual symptoms. I strongly suggest that you complete the self-evaluation exercises in this chapter when you first read it and once again after you have completed chapter 14, so you have a record of your growth and progress.

Chapter 8 is about the 7th chakra. Most chakra charts start at number 1, the root chakra at the base of the spine, and end with number 7, the crown chakra at the top of the head. I use the chakras in the opposite way, beginning with number 7. Chakra 7 is an overview, a way of looking at the whole person. When I conduct my readings, I begin here so that my guides can give me an overall summary of what the person may be facing and their root causes, rather than starting with specifics.

In chapter 8 and the rest of the chapters on the chakras, in addition to giving general "Call to Action" items that apply to every issue within that chakra, I discuss specific illnesses and conditions. My goal has been to offer information that is different from what you can find in other sources. Some issues and illnesses are covered more comprehensively than others, but the focus will always be to give information about root causes and healing.

Chapters 8 through 14 describe each section of the body in detail, organized by the chakras, along with their physical, emotional, and spiritual characteristics, a list of some corresponding illnesses and issues, and possible root causes. Each of these chapters also includes suggestions and tools you can use for resolving these issues and supporting wellness. The end of chapters 8–14 each has a list of questions you can reflect on yourself as well as ask your intuition, using the "Written Dialogue" technique (see chapter 5). This book includes specific advice and tools about intuitive eating, healing from trauma, spiritual development, body image, and individualized nutrition plans. I also provide specific information about practices that ameliorate specific chronic or severe illness that can be used to complement traditional medical protocols. I provide information about general health and wellness and tools for developing and understanding your empathic and psychic gifts. Throughout the book there are inspirational case studies from client experiences.

Part 2 is designed to be used as a glossary of conditions. It contains an index of specific physical, emotional, and spiritual conditions, arranged in alphabetical order, along with steps toward healing. The glossary is designed to provide additional information for healing, not to be a substitute for following the program for overall health and wellness. The appendix is a list of my favorite health and wellness–related websites, products, practitioners, techniques, and tools. I hope you find them as helpful as I do. The notes section contains links for studies and other information I have written about.

The tools and suggestions in this book can be used over and over again and can be applied to any illness or issue, now or in the future. As I recommended previously, you should evaluate yourself once as you begin this journey and again after completing chapter 14. The epilogue will give you suggestions for how to use the book in the future, when new issues or questions arise, or when you just want to check in with yourself to see how you are doing.

What I Believe

We cannot change anything unless we accept it.

—Carl Jung

- **With connection to intuition, self-love, and self-acceptance, we can heal from anything.**

I first learned this during my recovery from bulimia, and I believe it even more today thirty years later. We were born with self-love, and somewhere along the way were taught that we didn't deserve it, often by people who had been taught that they didn't deserve to love themselves. Part of illness and trauma often includes a wake-up call from our intuition to listen to our inner voices and to love and accept ourselves. To heal, it may be necessary to put ourselves first by setting healthy boundaries, expressing our opinions, and treating ourselves with respect. This emotional and spiritual part of recovery work can be frightening and more difficult than physical treatment and recovery, which is why people often avoid addressing these important root causes.

- **Excessive anxiety and thoughts about illness, trauma, and unhappiness can make healing more difficult.**

Our thoughts can become our reality. While in graduate school earning my special-education teaching certification, I learned about studies showing that when teachers raise the standards of their students and show them that they are capable of doing more challenging work, children's achievement is likely to increase as a result. If we tell ourselves that we cannot do something, we are basically guaranteeing it. Attitude can make the difference between success and failure.

This directly relates to the concept of being "a patient" and putting labels on ourselves. Of course, diagnoses are important so that practitioners can identify what is wrong and how to treat it. However, we are not our diagnoses, and we are certainly not defined by an illness or a disease. I have found that people are often negatively affected if their diagnosis becomes a part of their personality or identity. When I had Lyme disease, I was very careful not to use the word "Lyme" unless I absolutely had to, and not to use the word "my" in front of any symptoms or labels. I have learned not to say "my headache" or "my anxiety" or even "my problem." The issues are there and I acknowledge them, but I am not going to identify with them or let them become part of me. Positivity matters.

- **We cannot fully heal from emotional and physical issues unless we also address the spiritual root causes.**

This is why my readings are conducted on and about the whole person. Many of my clients begin the healing process believing that their physical or emotional issues don't run any deeper and are amazed at the progress we make once we start identifying and working on the spiritual issues in their life. They do not correlate headaches, achy joints, skin rashes, or the emergence of an autoimmune disease with their spouse's infidelity, death of a loved one, being in an abusive relationship, or taking care of a special-needs child. This is why I always ask what was going on in a person's life when their symptoms started, or if an accident happened. I haven't found many co-incidences.

Once these spiritual causes are identified and the client begins to take steps to address them, healing takes place at a much more rapid rate. If the client lets fear take over and stops addressing these issues, the symptoms often return or worsen.

· **Diagnosis and treatment must be individualized.**

Each of us is different, in terms of genetic makeup, gender, age, other conditions, medications and supplements we might be taking, belief systems, ability to detox and heal, and much more. In addition, one illness often takes on many different forms or severity and displays a wide variety of symptoms.

I have never been helped by one-size-fits-all protocols myself and have not found many clients who have been helped by them, either. I do not recommend them and do not use them.

· **If we push down our feelings and our intuition, especially trauma, they will later be expressed as physical and emotional symptoms. Symptoms are our intuition's way of getting our attention.**

In *The Body Keeps the Score*, Dutch psychiatrist Bessel van der Kolk writes about his research on trauma and the impact it has on physical, emotional, and spiritual aspects of health, including the physical symptoms expressed by survivors of trauma long after the incident occurred, and the transformational healing that happens once these survivors begin to allow themselves to feel what happened, tell others, and process it. He believes that talk therapy often isn't enough and that physical and symbolic methods of release must occur for true and lasting healing to take place.

Almost all clients who come to me with physical or mental health issues have underlying emotional or spiritual issues they are not aware of or are not allowing themselves to fully express. Many of the people I work with are trauma survivors who have done a great deal of work healing the trauma but are still holding fear, a lack of self-love, shame, or other feelings that they aren't even sure how to talk about. Their ultimate task is to move past the terrifying event(s) and live in the moment, rather than live in the past with the perceptions of how they used to be.

I can attest to the fact that our bodies express our emotions, especially ones that we have suppressed. It has happened to me many times, sometimes resulting in serious illness. This is the story of one of those times, when ignoring my feelings and intuition led to a year of mysterious, intense pain from a very bizarre source.

In addition to being a licensed counselor and medical intuitive, I am also a watercolor artist. From approximately 2002 to 2007, I was painting nearly every day. My work was in several galleries and prestigious national and international shows. I'd even had my own show at an esteemed New York City gallery, a dream come true.

If you have ever attempted to have creative thoughts during stressful times, you know this can be nearly impossible. In 2007, when my family was dealing with a great deal of stress, I stopped painting. I let the anxiety take over and crush my creativity. I lost all faith and contact with my intuition; I was a complete mess.

The abdominal pain and cramping began soon after. The intensity and frequency started slowly and built up until the pain would last for days at a time, coming on without warning. It was debilitating.

I lost track of how many MRIs, CT scans, and exams I had. Everything appeared to be "normal" and the doctors were baffled. Even after having my appendix removed, exploratory surgery, and discovering a rare type of cancerous tumor called a carcinoid, the pain persisted. After a year of nearly constant pain, my gynecologist was able to feel an abnormality with my uterus, and so we scheduled a hysterectomy.

Neither the doctor nor I were prepared for what she found.

My left fallopian tube and ovary had wrapped around my uterus, sticking to it. The uterus is the center of creativity. It is where life comes from. When I emotionally cut off my creativity and my spirituality, my body cut it off physically. It was a painful warning never to discontinue communication with my guides and intuition ever again and to never to let fear, despair, and feeling victimized take over.

This experience beautifully illustrates what I have come to believe. Rather than facing the difficult and painful emotions related to the stress my family and I were experiencing, I pushed the feelings down, choosing to believe that I wasn't strong enough to cope and that I was powerless. I blocked out my intuition and faith in God/Spirit, deciding instead to try to control the events and outcome, thinking that if they did not conform to my expectations, disaster would ensue. I pushed aside all of my previously effective problem solving and stress-relieving tools, allowing anxiety and depression to take over, which only intensified my symptoms. I lost faith in myself.

These responses are very common with stress and trauma. No one wants to dwell on fear, feeling helpless, sadness, or hurt, and we think that if we put it out of our heads, it either doesn't exist or will go away. The truth is that energy created by these emotions doesn't go away unless we bring those emotions to the surface and process them. Unless we find healthy ways to cope with difficulty, these feelings go into our bodies and are expressed as symptoms, but most people do not connect their physical symptoms with emotional or spiritual pain.

When you are faced with situations that are beyond your control, you may feel helpless, but since this just brings on additional anxiety, you may do anything to try to numb yourself. The best approach is to allow yourself to feel that pain and *think* logically about what you can do. Feel your emotions, but don't allow yourself to be consumed by them; instead, begin to problem-solve. Don't take situations personally, assuming that difficult things are happening because you are "being punished," are a bad person, or that it is just karma. Ask yourself how you can learn from the situation and make different choices next time, or how you could better listen to the warning signals from your intuition.

My story is unique to me, but it illustrates the universal principles I've discussed in this chapter. Most importantly, it shows a path toward healing. When one-size-fits-all diagnoses and treatments fail, it's an invitation to listen deeply to our intuition and bodies, to accept what they are telling us without judgment or anger, and to begin making the choices that will lead to healing.

REFLECTIONS ON CHAPTER 2

- What are your coping mechanisms for stress, if any?
- Did you have positive role models for dealing with painful situations?
- Can you think of times when stress and trauma resulted in physical and emotional symptoms?
- What are some strategies for dealing with fear and other difficult feelings during a situation you cannot control, such as losing someone close to you or experiencing a natural disaster?
- Can you recall times in your life when you tried to control a situation according to your agenda, only to realize later that things worked out for the best when you let go?

Finding My Life Purpose

One looks back with appreciation to the brilliant teachers, but with gratitude to those who touched our human feelings.

—Carl Jung

I still vividly remember the day I started to release my fear and allow my authentic self to emerge, with the help of what I am convinced is divine intervention. This was the first time I felt truly connected to my intuition and decided to trust it, though I had no idea that was what I was doing at the time.

It was winter during my senior year in high school, and I was struggling with bulimia. I had also recently found out that I received a scholarship to George Washington University. The thought of being able to move away from my parents and live six hours from my dysfunctional homelife in Connecticut was exciting and gave me hope for the future. I hadn't felt hopeful in a very long time.

I'm not sure exactly what gave me the courage, but I came home from school one day and picked up the yellow rotary wall phone in the kitchen, my hands shaking as I dialed the number of our family pediatrician, Dr. Merman. When I told him that I was eating a lot and throwing up three times a day, he initially said that he thought I would be fine, that it wasn't any cause for concern. In 1983, not very much was known about eating disorders. I even used the word "bulimic," which I had never done before. I had never been so afraid to make a phone call in my entire life, and I'm so thankful that whatever gave me the courage and motivation to call also made me fight to make sure that he listened to me. I didn't tell him that if he didn't give me the name of a therapist, I was considering ending my life by driving my car into a wall. I thought he might tell my parents, who would put me into a hospital, and then everyone would find out how really screwed up I was. Fortunately, he took what I was saying seriously and gave me the name of a therapist: Jean Sutherland, a licensed clinical social worker, who was trained in Jungian psychology.

Two months after making that call, after repeatedly telling myself that I could stop on my own, I mustered up the courage to phone the therapist he recommended. She asked if my parents would be coming, and I said, "No, just me. Is that okay?" When she said that I was old enough to receive treatment on my own, I was so relieved. There was no way I could explain what I had been doing to myself or the incomprehensible thoughts in my head, in front of the people I knew had contributed to my eating disorder and who would deny any responsibility, much less make any effort to change their behavior.

The only time I felt really recognized by my father was when I gained or lost weight. I hadn't even noticed the twenty pounds I gained after going through puberty at age twelve, until my father made a comment that I "didn't need" the ice cream I was getting out of the freezer. Sitting in judgment at the kitchen table, with his ever-present large belly, he was hardly someone who should be giving nutritional advice. I didn't say very much (and never did then), dishing myself a few scoops anyway, but I secretly vowed to start dieting the next day. By the end of that summer, taking in only a thousand calories a day (because why do anything in moderation?), I had lost all of the weight I had gained. Soon after, I returned to my normal way of eating and gained it all back, starting a vicious cycle of gain and loss.

As the number on the scale increased, I spiraled deeper into the pattern of self-hatred and failure, and the weight loss became even more difficult with the damage I was doing to my metabolism. Eventually, I resorted to desperate measures: first bingeing and fasting on and off for days at a time, using laxatives and diuretics. When these "weight loss" methods didn't work, I turned to bulimia. I ate more during the binges than I threw up, so I didn't lose weight doing that, either, but by then it wasn't about the weight. It was about trying to push down my feelings. It had become a full-blown addiction.

Bingeing and purging is a way of removing yourself from your body, going to a different place, where there are no feelings, other people, pressures—anything. It's an escape from real life and from yourself. It's a way of letting go of all control, expectations, and fears—saying "fuck you" to life with the binge, then vomiting up that temporary courage. I was ready to find lasting courage.

On my first day of therapy, I had what I can only describe as an out-of-body experience. I felt the presence of a force that had always been a part of me but that I never recognized. It was an inner strength and an inner love. It was making me fight and telling me I could win. It was telling me that I could beat this.

The concepts my therapist described were completely foreign to me. I had never heard of Carl Jung or Jungian psychology, the collective unconscious, archetypes, the Shadow, alchemy, or most of the other things the therapist talked about, but I loved that our work was based on connection to intuition, acceptance of the whole person, and self-love. I loved that Jung developed the majority of his most important teachings and theories during active trance states in which he communicated in writing and through artistic images with his intuitive guides. They are based on and have influenced mythology, archaeology, religion, art, astrology, anthropology, and the occult. His views and the tools he created made sense to me, since they encouraged empowerment, connection to intuition, and the belief that we already have the answers to our problems and questions inside of ourselves. I just needed guidance to help find them.

I inhaled everything my therapist gave me to read and attended appointments every week until I went off to college that fall. While I was engaging in eating-disordered behaviors less and less, I still had a long way to go emotionally. I continued with therapy at school, and within a couple of years, I had stopped the bingeing and purging and other eating-disordered behaviors completely, but the desire and body dysmorphia (seeing your body differently than the way it actually looks) remained. I was prescribed the antidepressant Prozac toward the end of my therapy. Knowing what I know now, I may not have chosen that route, but at that time it truly changed my life for the better. I became less sensitive, saw myself and life through a clearer lens, and became much more outgoing. As an added bonus, I no longer felt the desire to engage in bulimic behavior.

WHAT IS A MEDICAL INTUITIVE?

In 1989, I finished graduate school with a master's in counseling, eventually getting my license. Most of my career has been spent in private practice, but I have also worked with children and adolescents for a community service organization, been an art therapist, a counselor for private companies in day treatment and residential facilities, and a drug counselor with adults involved in dual diagnosis (people with both mental illness and addiction) programs. I went back to college and earned a certification in special education and school psychology and worked in schools in both Virginia and Connecticut.

I have always been what you would call an "eclectic" therapist, using whatever techniques were most appropriate to the

individual, but my approach has been strongly based on Jungian psychology, and I *always* listen to my intuition for guidance. The very best sessions were the ones where I felt I was
almost "out of body" and my guides were right there with me.

The more I worked with people and relied on my guides, the
more "unusual" but incredibly natural experiences occurred.
I knew things about clients that they never told me, saw situations, people, and places in my head that hadn't been shared, and
would say things my clients were thinking. To be honest, I wasn't
entirely comfortable with my abilities and didn't know what to
do with them, but I knew that I needed to embrace and use them.
I just wasn't sure how.

One of these experiences that made me take my abilities
more seriously was when I worked with a young woman in her
late twenties who suffered from bulimia. She and her husband
had been trying to get pregnant for a very long time. Although
pregnancy while actively eating disordered can be extremely
dangerous for the mother and baby, she was making progress
in her treatment.

I was teaching her the technique I will later teach you, which
is to have a dialogue with her intuition. She wasn't understanding the concept, so I asked her to name a special person in her
life she could talk to instead of her intuition. She talked about
her cherished and greatly missed grandmother, who had passed
away when she was young. I offered to do a role-play and "be"
her grandmother to demonstrate how to use the technique.

Much to my surprise, I immediately began seeing images of
her grandmother in my head, like photos in a picture frame. As
we went on with the exercise, I started to see images of the attic
where she played in her grandmother's house as a child, and her
favorite doll. I shared all of this with her and described her grandmother. I knew things she had never told anyone. We were both in
a bit of shock at my accuracy. Her grandmother (through me) said
that she wanted her to have a child and that she was going to help.

About eight weeks later, the young woman reported that

she was pregnant and that conception had taken place shortly after our appointment. For the first time, I realized that my intuitive and psychic-medium abilities could be valuable tools, and I started to work on actively developing them. The only people I really talked to about them were my husband, my grandmother, my therapist (when seeing one), and occasionally my mother. I had never felt comfortable opening up to anyone else.

A couple of years later, in 2010, a friend told me about a Spiritualist church near my house, and I attended the first service reluctantly, not knowing what to expect. When I heard the minister use the words "medium readings" and "hands-on healing," I knew I was home.

As I became involved in the church, I started exploring my gift for the first time, taking evidential mediumship classes with some of the nicest, most giving people I had ever met, who had been practicing it for decades. Instead of being judgmental or skeptical, the church leadership encouraged my gifts, and I found the courage to get up in front of the congregation and did a few, quite accurate, group readings. I was finally leaning into my gifts and finding my place.

But less than a year later, my life would be turned upside-down.

In December of 2008, as a result of a flu shot, my previously healthy mother became suddenly paralyzed over 90 percent of her body and legally blind. She spent the next ten years in this state, gradually getting worse and passing away. During the first four years, I was her caretaker, with my husband's support, and I was also her power of attorney and health-care agent. It was a twenty-four seven job managing her care and treatment. As anyone who has been in a similar situation knows, especially when dysfunctional family dynamics are involved, it's common for power struggles, sibling rivalry, and much worse to occur. Countless police, doctors, nurses, social workers, psychiatrists, judges, and other experienced professionals told me that the conduct of my family, with the exception of my husband and daughters, was some of the most dysfunctional and destructive they had ever encountered.

This experience changed me dramatically. I had a new perspective on what was truly important and what were just "small things." Life can be taken away in a fraction of a second, so it is vital to cherish what you have and be grateful. I had to come to terms with some hard truths about my family and came to realize that the relationships I thought were loving had not been. I learned who truly cared and who never really had. The end of these toxic relationships is one of the best things that came out of my mother's illness and something that should have happened long before it did.

It was impossible to go back to how my life was before this happened. I wasn't the same person. Even the therapy work and painting I had been doing didn't seem to be as meaningful. I was truly ready to be myself and not let what others thought or said get in my way. I just didn't know what that meant.

That changed when I found out about a workshop on medical intuition given by a well-known medical intuitive at the Omega Institute for Holistic Studies in Rhinebeck, New York. I wasn't exactly sure what medical intuition was, but the idea of working with the physical body and intuition seemed fascinating, and I signed up immediately. The medical intuitive opened the workshop by giving us the names of persons and their ages and telling us to write down everything we knew, saw, or heard about the subjects. I was afraid that nothing would come to mind. However, to my amazement, I started seeing images of the person's (or animal's) body with great detail, both inside and out, knowing things about their childhoods and emotional characteristics, feeling their exact emotions and more. By the end of the first day, I knew I had found my calling.

As I learned more about medical intuition, I developed my own methods and eventually started working one-on-one with clients. This is my way of using my gifts, listening to my intuition, and helping people who are deeply hurting.

If I hadn't separated from my toxic family, I may have let their judgmental criticism keep me from pursuing my dreams. Painful as it was, coming to terms with how destructive my family was freed me to follow my intuition and find my life path. I never felt comfortable enough with any of them to reveal my authentic self. All of the traumatic and stressful experiences I have had, which seemed so horrible at the time, brought their own gifts. I have been transformed from a timid, depressed, overweight, addicted, self-destructive adolescent with post-traumatic stress disorder to a brave, healthy, incredibly strong, determined, happy person. When I started therapy, I was convinced that no one would ever love me or think I was beautiful. I have been married to my husband for more than twenty-five years and couldn't ask for a more supportive or loving person to share my life with. Together, we have raised two amazing, accomplished young women with honesty, acceptance, encouragement, and stability—completely the opposite of how I was raised.

These transformations are possible for you too, no matter how impossible that may seem. You wouldn't be reading this book if at least some part of you didn't believe that you could be happy and healthy. At times, for me, it was two steps forward and one step back, but that is how we learn. Healing does not happen in a linear fashion. This book will help you determine what you need to do and give you the courage to take the first steps.

I am truly blessed and I am excited to be part of the start of your new life.

My Unique, Individual Reading Process

The shoe that fits one person pinches another; there is no recipe for living that suits all cases.

—Carl Jung

The goals of my readings are to identify and help heal the root physical, spiritual, and emotional causes of problems and symptoms, strengthen communication with intuition, teach unconditional love and acceptance, and provide a guide for how to live authentically. When I conduct a reading, I give specific tools and guidance about nutrition, recommend people look into specific supplements, explore healthy creativity and other stress-relieving outlets, examine their relationships and self-care, and teach them how to problem solve.

I also help people find practitioners who can verify what I have picked up, do appropriate testing, administer (hopefully) holistic treatments if possible, and more. I try to recommend only practitioners whom I have worked and communicated with.

I conducted research about my abilities and accuracy for an article published several years ago in the *International Journal of Healing and Caring*. I sent seventy-five of my former clients, as well as some of their physicians (with their permission), a questionnaire along with the report I had created for them when we worked together. I asked them their opinion on the reading, my accuracy, and how many of the details (which I numbered on the report) were correct. They rated my accuracy at 97 percent.

I am often asked how I can be so accurate, especially considering that I create my reports and paintings knowing only a name and age, before ever meeting with a client, seeing a photo, or receiving any information from them except an email and phone number. The information is extremely personal and detailed, with more than seventy-five specific facts initially revealed before our meeting, and more during our time together.

Before I discovered that I have spiritual guides, I described the information I received about myself and others as coming from my intuition. It is perfectly okay if you do not connect with "guides," and I often use the word "intuition" interchangeably with the word "guides." The label isn't important, just that you listen. I believe that we all have guides, angels, loved ones who have passed, and higher beings who watch over us, love us, and send us information we need to be happy and healthy. The same techniques I will teach you later to connect with your intuition and body can also be used to connect with your guides.

Since I am often asked about them, I will talk a little about what I experience when working with my guides. When I visualize them, I sometimes see a table in the shape of a semicircle, with me in the middle and many people seated around it. I have been told I have an "army" of guides. We all do. I don't know the names of my guides, except for my maternal grandparents and my mother, who are in spirit. As for the others, I have seen some of them in meditations and know that they are male and female. I have never seen their faces clearly, and they are not always the same people. I know that they are connected with God, which to me is pure, true love, more powerful than any evil or negativity. I don't know how my guides come up with the information (it isn't me personally) or how it can be so accurate. I wish I could explain it, but I wouldn't even know where to start.

Knowing only a client's name and age, before seeing a photo or exchanging any specifics, with information downloaded from my guides I create a detailed, four-page report and a symbolic painting. I use the chakras—the seven major energy centers in the body—as a framework for my report and readings. The report contains two columns at the top, one labeled "Emotional" and one labeled "Physical," with a section for each chakra. The report format helps me organize my ideas and gives people descriptions of the chakras as well as written information about what I initially hear from my guides. I will be teaching you how to create a similar report of your own that you can use to heal and grow.

The paintings I create are an extension of my love of art, art therapy, and symbolism. They explore the power of nonverbal expression and provide a different way for clients to see and process the information. Even though they look like a toddler created them, they are incredibly powerful, and many clients even frame them. I am excited to teach you how to create your own intuitive paintings.

My readings and the techniques and methods described in this book are all based on the chakras. Chakras have been described by Eastern religions for centuries as points of connection between the physical and spiritual body. They are vertically aligned from the base of the spine (root chakra) to the crown on the top of the head (crown chakra).

Ideally, as we grow up, we work through the lessons in each chakra, from root to crown, and progress from the material, basic needs like food, clothing, shelter, physical and emotional safety, etc. (1st chakra); to relationships, sexuality, and finances (2nd chakra); to self-esteem and personality (3rd chakra); to processing emotions and caring for others (4th chakra); to will, authenticity, and self-expression (5th chakra); to intellect, intuition, and insight (6th chakra); and finally to connection to the Divine (7th chakra).

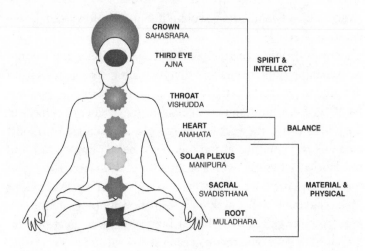

If we fail to learn these lessons or if we succumb to fear that keeps us from developing and growing because of physical or emotional trauma, illness, or a host of other issues, the energy flow through the body, or "chi" as it's called in Chinese medicine, is disrupted. When this happens, we risk becoming stuck and creating physical, emotional, and spiritual illness. Energy healing works, among other reasons, because it restores the balance of the chakras and the energy flow within and around the body. Disruption in one chakra impacts all of the others.

My readings address these energy disruptions. They're incredibly thorough and contain information about every chakra and every aspect of a client's life, not only including physical symptoms and root causes but also emotional and spiritual ones. I delve into people's childhood experiences, work life, family, traumas, abilities, life purpose, fears and expectations, belief systems, and more, which I will address in detail in future chapters. Everything my guides tell me is considered and passed on. This is the same powerful, soul-deep exploration you will be learning to do in chapter 7.

The report shown here is one I used with an actual patient. I clear my mind and ask that the reading be for the client's highest and best good. I then choose an oracle card for the client from one of my decks to get me out of my own head and start the process. I write down a short description of the message from the card and give my interpretation.

Next to the descriptions is the information I received from my guides regarding the client's physical and emotional characteristics, spiritual life, intuitive and psychic ability, relationships, self-esteem, family history, professional life, and so on.

Emotional		Physical	
7TH CHAKRA		**7TH CHAKRA**	
(Crown) Purpose in life, relationship with spirit	I feel like you have had a strong relationship with yourself, strong faith and relationship with your intuition. I feel some distance or blocks lately and like you have been questioning yourself as well as some of the advice you have been getting.	Life-threatening illnesses, chronic illnesses, brain, nervous system	Hearing that you have been feeling fatigued with inflammation, discomfort, pain. Also hearing that you take pretty good care of yourself and that you know what to do on many levels, so in some areas, you just need fine-tuning.
6TH CHAKRA		**6TH CHAKRA**	
(Third eye) Perception, thought, morality, flexibility, ability to change and blend in psychic ability	Hearing that you are a perceptive person and that you have strong third eye ability, with a good ability to judge the sincerity of people. Morality is important to you and you treat others the way you want to be treated. You pick up energies of people and spirits and always have but you may not have always been able to talk about this with others.	Head, nose, ears, anxiety, etc., pituitary gland, making and storing of hormones, pineal gland	Sensitive to chemicals, medications, mold, temperature extremes. Some anxiety. Strong sense of smell and sinus symptoms more frequently than you would like. Deviated septum. You are treating sinus symptoms currently and have in the past.

Emotional		Physical	
5TH CHAKRA		**5TH CHAKRA**	
(Throat) Self-expression, will, pushing forward vs. just waiting for things to happen, communication, activism in the world, voice	You are selective about who you share your feelings with and who you spend your time with. You would rather have quality, meaningful conversations with people you care about than just "small talk." You would like to have more people you could share your feelings with who would really listen. You haven't always expressed how you felt in the past and can be rather quiet. Wishing you had done some significant things differently and taken different opportunities.	Throat, mouth, teeth, thyroid, neck	Feeling some soreness in the throat and some energy blockage. Acid reflux. Thyroid likely sluggish; may have some Hashimoto's or could be from adrenal imbalance. Neck feels stiff but delicate at the same time. Are you able to chew the way you need to? I feel like you may not have all of your teeth and may need serious dental work or replacement or have had it done.
4TH CHAKRA		**4TH CHAKRA**	
(Heart) Emotions, intimacy, nurturance, partnership, giving vs. getting help, trust issues in relationships, care of others	Quite sensitive, empathic, and able to pick up the feelings of others and of animals. You have been able to pick up the feelings of people from a young age, and that could make life difficult at times. You have given more in some relationships than you have gotten back, and you have experienced significant hurt. Needing intimacy. Lifelong caretaker.	Heart, lungs, blood pressure, cholesterol, breasts	Your heart and cardio-vascular system may not be as healthy as it should be, and I also feel like your heart is sad. It feels like your heart is working very hard. Any blockages, plaque buildup, or things like that you are aware of? Breathing feels shallow and like you may forget to breathe. Ever a smoker or exposed to smoke?

Emotional		Physical	
3RD CHAKRA		**3RD CHAKRA**	
(Solar plexus) Self-esteem, fulfill responsibility to self and others, discipline, care of self	Overall you feel pretty good about yourself but that you can be excessively hard on yourself at times and struggle with perfectionism. You have a need for control, and sometimes it is hard to relax and let go. You are much better at this than you used to be, though. You take your responsibilities seriously but can also have fun. Lately, not as much fun as you would like.	Small intestine, stomach, addictions, liver, adrenal hormones, blood sugar, gallbladder, kidneys, spleen	Your gut feels like it is out of balance and like it has been affected by medications. Feeling some food intolerances, like dairy, perhaps histamines. Adrenal fatigue. Liver feels a bit clogged, not that it would show up on any tests. Blood sugar feels like it can get both high and low, like you sometimes forget to eat, but that when you do, you go for high-sugar and high-carb foods.
2ND CHAKRA		**2ND CHAKRA**	
(Sacral) Balancing relationships vs. money, you and I vs. we, creativity	You feel separate from people you care about, maybe "distanced" is a more appropriate word. You feel emotionally distant in some cases and geographically distant in others, perhaps both in some. Grieving and sadness. You are a creative person, but you don't make enough time for it and don't try new things because you don't think you will be good at them.	Reproductive organs, bladder, prostate, large intestine, lower back	From my guides hearing dryness and discomfort. In the past it feels like you had issues with some cell growth, like endometriosis or fibroids. Pain, in your uterus or other organs. Perhaps being in uncomfortable positions. Lower back pain.

Emotional		Physical	
1ST CHAKRA		**1ST CHAKRA**	
(Root) Family issues, belonging, trust, safety and security, caretaking vs. being a loner vs. being wishy-washy, basic needs	The first thing I heard here was, again, loss and grieving. Major loss affected important relationships or a main relationship. Never really got over it. Guilt, even though it is misplaced. Relied on yourself emotionally in childhood. You did have people who loved and cared for you, though. Hearing alcoholism or substance abuse in immediate family.	Base of spine, blood, joints, bones, immune system, lymph system, allergies, skin	Picking up inflammation, joint pain, muscle aches. Sleep issues. Bone density. Immune system, vitamin D likely an issue. Skin feels fair and sensitive. Allergies. Hearing about some possible underlying viral activity and fibromyalgia-type symptoms or similar issues.

Over the course of your work with this book, you'll be able to create a chart like this one for yourself as you learn to tap into your intuition to identify different issues.

After finishing the report, I create a watercolor painting symbolizing the body, energy, and "aura" of the client. Aura is the energy and light field that surrounds every living thing. It can be in the form of a figure, an animal, plant life, or whatever else my guides choose to use to illustrate their message. Every painting is very different. To begin, I usually see or hear a color, then create the image. Sometimes I show energy being released or needing to be released; sometimes I show energy that is blocked. Everything is significant, from the positioning of the arms, the size of the shoulders, the directions the feet are facing, the colors themselves and their positioning, whether the body is touching the ground or not, etc. Finally, I make written notes on the painting and send the report and painting to the clients several hours before our meeting.

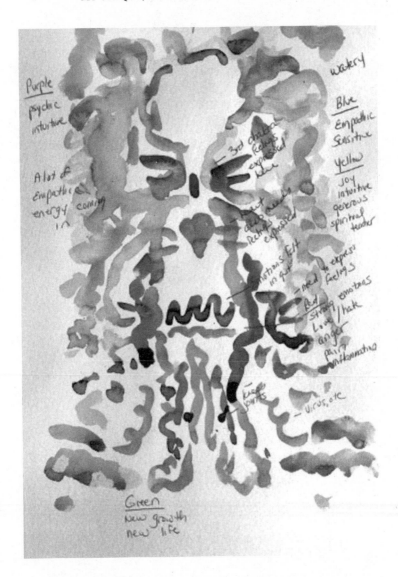

This is an example of an intuitive painting. Flip to the front and back of the book to see other paintings reproduced on the endpapers.

This book is designed to empower you to use many of these same techniques to explore and address the areas of your life that need healing. We are all guided by intuition, even if we don't recognize it. The challenging part can be learning to listen to it and trust it, especially if we grew up in an environment or culture that didn't teach us how.

You Are Never Alone

Connecting to Intuition

Who looks outside, dreams; who look inside awakes.

—Carl Jung

One of the most common reasons people reach out to me is because they feel like their intuition is blocked. They think that they cannot listen, that they overthink the process, or that they simply don't have any intuitive abilities. Once I teach them my techniques for connecting to their intuition and how to develop confidence in themselves and the process, they are amazed at how easy it can be and how dramatically their lives can change.

When the idea of connecting to intuition was first proposed to me as a path to recovery from bulimia, I couldn't imagine how it would help me let go of my addiction to bingeing and purging or help me to lose weight, which I mistakenly thought would solve all of my problems. I barely even knew what intuition was, and I certainly didn't think I was going to be successful at recovery. But I was committed and desperate, willing to try just about anything that might help me heal. I never dreamed that intuition would save my life and that someday I would teach people all over the world to follow their own.

My definition of intuition, borrowed from Carl Jung and

shared with me by my first Jungian therapist, Jean Sutherland, is simply "God within."

Intuition isn't just about predicting what will happen in the future or being able to tell people things about themselves that they didn't tell you. It is so much more than that. It is an all-knowing, all-powerful force that is part of all of us and all living things. It is pure love. It always keeps us safe and loves and accepts us unconditionally. I sometimes describe it as being like a pet who loves you without any judgment.

Intuition knows what is best for you, even when you do not. It is like the perfect parent or bodyguard who is always there guiding and supporting you. Once I found my intuition, I never felt alone or unsafe again.

OBSTACLES TO CONNECTING TO INTUITION

As you first begin tuning in to your intuition, it's normal to wonder if you are listening to your intuition, or fear, or yourself. "I don't feel any different"; "I don't hear anything"; "I want to see colors or pictures"; "the voice sounds just like mine"; and "I want exact answers"—these are points often brought up by clients who don't think they can connect.

The voice I hear when I'm talking to my intuition sounds just like mine, but sometimes it feels like it comes from a deeper place or somewhere from outside of myself. When I'm asking for information during readings and learning about a client, I just let what I hear fill the page and don't question it. I've been doing it long enough and have enough faith in my accuracy to know that I can trust it, but that takes time. If I am distracted by anxiety or things I need to do, I know that I have to push that aside or my accuracy will be in jeopardy.

In my own work, I am able to see colors, words, symbols, people, scenes, feel physical sensations, and hear words. But I haven't always been able to. These are skills I've developed over time as I learn to pay closer attention to my intuition. I have medium abilities, so I can communicate with people who have passed. I can also pick up knowledge by touching people and objects. It makes sense that I would have all of these abilities, since I use them every day and this work is my life purpose, but if you don't, that doesn't mean that your own personal intuitive or psychic abilities are any less valid or strong. Your intuition is all-knowing and all-powerful, and as you continue to develop your own ability to listen to it, you will find that the messages you receive will be clearer and more detailed.

These are some common obstacles people encounter when trying to listen to their intuition:

- **Attempting to control the message you receive:** You may not want to hear what you are told, and it isn't uncommon for intuition to tell you something unrelated to what you are asking about. Be open to the possibilities.

- **Self-doubt and overthinking:** You will not always be accurate or on target. That is okay. Perhaps it won't seem accurate at the time, but it may later prove to be.

- **Asking questions about the future, especially about things that have yet to be determined:** An example might be, "Who will I marry?" or "What state will I live in in ten years?" or "How many children will I have?" You may get an answer, but often these can be frustrating questions because our intuition wants us to experience life and make mistakes, not just know what is going to happen.

- **Asking questions that are too vague or complicated:** For instance, "What is my life purpose?" There are so many possible answers because we have many life purposes.

- **Believing that you must act on what you learn immediately:** People in bad relationships or jobs usually know that they have to leave, but they may not know how or might not be ready. You can be open to the information without having to act on it. Your intuition gives you possibilities and ideas; it doesn't force you to do anything. You have free will.

- **Believing that if you aren't seeing colors, hearing voices, or having a "mystical experience," you haven't done it right:** Although I've had amazing spiritual experiences, I would definitely not call the majority of my personal spiritual interactions "mystical." The quiet whisper of intuition is just as powerful as technicolor vision.

- **Believing that you aren't intuitive:** Some people fear that if they aren't mediums, psychics, medical intuitives, or people with "special" recognized abilities, they must not be intuitive. We all have the ability to connect with intuition.

- **General anxiety, trauma, or anything that prevents you from being in the present moment:** If you are always thinking about the past or the future, you cannot be grounded in the present. This is essential for being able to listen.

- **Blocking out feelings:** If you can't listen to your feelings, you definitely can't be open to listening to intuition.

- **Not being connected to the body:** This might be because of emotional or physical pain, poor body image, body dysmorphia, eating disorders, sexual assault, or abuse. The body is an important source of intuitive information, since intuition uses symptoms to get our attention.

- **Lack of sleep:** If you are tired and irritable, it is difficult to focus on anything, much less intuition.

- **Fear of connecting with negative or evil forces:** This can dramatically block your ability to connect with your intuition. Most people think that if they open up to loving intuitive or spiritual forces, they will automatically open up to the dangerous ones as well, but this isn't true. I'm not saying that evil doesn't exist; it does, and it would like nothing better than to keep us from talking with our loving intuition and with other forces that connect us with God, the universe, and love. It uses fear to trick us into thinking that we are not safe and that it's lurking over our shoulders, ready to pounce once we let our guard down. I used to think this was true, and for a long time it made me turn away from my abilities and amazing life-giving intuitive connection.

Regarding the last point, I believe that *you and you alone are in control of your energy.* If you are tuned in to love, you cannot be harmed. Love is always more powerful than hate, evil, and fear. There are a few situations in which you may not be in total control of your energy, and those are during states of addiction (altered consciousness) or when you have *willingly* opened yourself up to negative energy and negative people. You must choose whom you allow into your world. If you feel negativity, it is important that you remove yourself from the situation and the influence of those people.

Being in the presence of evil or negative people does not allow them to take over or exert power over you. That is up to you, but it can happen over time without you realizing it. I have seen it happen to those I know very well. People who once had good hearts turned against their children, family, and friends because of the manipulative influences of angry, negative, and evil people.

I have learned that we can never be touched by evil or negativity if we have love in our hearts. Your intuition is defined by unconditional love, and you should never be afraid to listen to it. I touch on this more in future chapters.

Most kids can feel spirits and even pick up the energy of people who have passed. Many later forget because they had no one to talk to about it or they were too afraid, both of which were the case for me. When I was nine or ten years old, I recall feeling significant amounts of evil in my home. I was constantly terrified, like something was after me, trying to hurt me, and I knew I had to be vigilant to fight it off and protect myself. The fear associated with picking up negative entities, people, and energy can cause us to fear our intuitive and psychic abilities as a whole, and that is exactly what happened to me. I blocked them out until I began therapy for bulimia.

My therapist taught me that fear of evil was perfectly acceptable and real. Many people don't take evil and negativity seriously, but I know that evil exists, and that is why I was so frightened. I learned that I was the one with the power, not any outside forces, and that I could protect myself. This is a critical lesson for everyone looking to explore their intuition: you hold the power, and no evil force can change that.

CONNECTING WITH AND STRENGTHENING INTUITION

TECHNIQUE ONE: WRITTEN DIALOGUE

There are many techniques for connecting with and strengthening intuition. My favorite, and the one I find most effective, is what I call Written Dialogue.

This is not a formal exercise and does not require a large time commitment. I have a journal that I write in every morning for usually ten to twenty minutes, but I've also been known to write for five minutes on a napkin in my car. You don't have to do this exercise daily, but the more you use it, the greater the connection will be.

You will be directing this exercise to your intuition, which you could also call God, your higher self, your guides, etc.— whatever makes the most sense to you. You can, and I encourage you to, use this to talk to your body, your illness, and people who have passed as well. At first, you may find it helpful to do a short meditation, take a walk, or engage in a creative activity before beginning to write in order to clear your head and distract you from thinking about daily to-do lists and responsibilities.

To begin:

1. Write down a question or your feelings and direct it to your intuition, God, or whatever you wish to communicate with. Be confident you will receive an answer.
2. Write down what you immediately hear. Be sure to note answers that may not be conveyed in words. What do you feel in response, both physically and emotionally, to the question?
3. Write a response to what you heard or felt. As in a typical conversation, your response might be a further question, a comment, or a whole new line of enquiry.
4. Listen for any comment, question, etc. related to what you wrote in step 3, and write down what you hear, feel, or sense in answer.
5. Respond in writing.
6. Continue the conversation for as long as you like.

Pay special attention to the list of obstacles discussed earlier in this chapter when you begin this practice. At first, you may only hear a single word, but don't be afraid to ask for more information. The more you do it, the easier it will become. There is no right or wrong way to do this exercise or any required amount of time to spend on it. Sometimes I write for a considerable length of time, and sometimes I scratch out a few sentences. Do whatever feels comfortable for you. You'll find suggestions for "Intuitive Writing Prompts" listed at the beginning of each chakra chapter (8–14).

Sometimes I just start writing about an event in my life, as I would if I were discussing it with a friend, and ask my intuition for feedback or guidance. If I am feeling sad or anxious but don't know why, I will just start writing down random thoughts, like a stream of consciousness, and ask for guidance. I also ask direct questions like these: "What feelings have I been pushing down?" "What am I afraid of?" "Is there anything you would like to tell me today?" "How can I be more authentic?" "Should I do this or that?" If you ask a yes-or-no question, follow it up by asking for more information. I don't suggest asking questions about the future, like "Will that happen?" or "When will this happen?" because that is a way to try to predict the future. We often ask these sorts of questions when we are afraid of living in the present moment and are trying to avoid making important decisions using our own intuition.

As I mentioned, you might receive a response that doesn't seem to fit or is about a different topic. That is because your intuition (or whomever or whatever you are writing to) has something else that is important to tell you.

For example, you may ask a question and hear "Stop." You're probably being guided to stop thinking or worrying about what you wanted to know. If you do not receive an answer, it may not be an appropriate question or be one that you necessarily need an answer to. Try asking something else, or ask your intuition what it would like you to know.

Don't be afraid to be honest. Your intuition isn't going to get mad and reject you. If you are angry, express that. Be yourself. Your intuition loves and accepts you. Let it be a source of love and comfort. Trust that it knows what is best for you.

It is important to do this exercise *in writing* and not just in your head. When you do, it becomes a form of mindfulness meditation because you have to stop what you are doing and focus on writing. You are less likely to be distracted by the many thoughts of the day if your hand is occupied with kinesthetic activity. As you do this exercise, pay attention to what the intuitive voice sounds and feels like. It may come from a certain direction or settle in certain parts of the body. You may see words or images. You may feel things physically. Take it all in and write it down. The more you practice, the easier it is and the more you will be able to recognize your intuition all the time, not just when you are doing this exercise.

When I first used this exercise to talk to my body and my bulimia, it was a game changer. I talked to them as my friends instead of my enemies. I still view the eating disorder as one of the best things that ever happened to me. I now think of it as a friend who came along to help me separate from my dysfunctional family, heal trauma and negative thinking, find self-love and authenticity, and made me realize that I was not a victim. Seeing my body as something that needed love, care, and respect, instead of constant criticism, abuse, and hatred, was something I never dreamed would occur.

When I help clients learn these techniques and see their relationships with themselves and their bodies transform, it is incredibly gratifying.

TECHNIQUE TWO: INTUITIVE SOUL PAINTING

Intuitive Soul Painting is a technique I developed that I use during each of my intuitive readings. It is a symbolic representation of the body, the energy around the body, and someone's emotional and spiritual states. Just like the report, it can reflect both present day and the past. There is a black-and-white example of one of these in chapter 4, and color examples in the endpapers of this book and my website, www .katiebeecher.com.

Anyone can create these paintings; no artistic ability is required. These are not polished masterpieces, but raw, unedited creations that reflect emotion, energy, and Spirit through color and form.

I consider these paintings an essential part of my work. Unlike the information in a written report, which we can more easily misinterpret with our humanness, the information in the paintings is completely symbolic. It can be tempting to interpret what we hear or write from our guides to the point where we are no longer listening. The painting resists any kind of conscious or unconscious manipulation. As you begin painting (or creating in another medium you choose), you'll discover that this is a powerful way to deepen your connection with intuition without being restricted by conscious thought and overanalyis. Art helps intuition speak in a new way.

When you create a piece of intuitive art, I don't want you to think about purposely creating any symbolic meaning. You will not immediately understand the context of what you've created. When I paint, no cognition is involved. The vast majority of the time, I don't know the meanings of the symbols and placement of the colors until I discuss the painting with my client and get new information from my guides as we explore the essence of the piece.

The images I create are all different and are usually human figures, but I have painted flowers and plants, animals, trees, buildings, and even a fire truck, which was one of my most memorable paintings.

I created it several years ago when doing a reading for a five-year-old boy with severe autism. I knew only his name and age when I started the reading. After completing the report, I saw a clear image of a fire truck and a building in my mind. As I was trying to paint the hose on the side of the fire truck, I remember having difficulty rendering it. I kept thinking that it just looked like a giant "S," and I said to myself that my client will think it is Superman's fire truck.

When I described the painting for his mother, I told her that the "S" on the side was supposed to be a fire hose and I joked that I thought she would think it belonged to Superman. At that point, she began to cry. She explained that the year before she became pregnant with her son, the apartment she lived in was destroyed by a fire and she lost everything. She lost hope and was ready to end her life, until she found out that she was pregnant.

Her son brought her back to life and gave her a reason to

move forward. She believed that her son was a gift who would bring many people joy, not only her. She called him her "Superman," even giving him Superman's middle name, Joseph. This painting was a confirmation of everything she had come to believe.

This is the power of intuitive art. Even a detail as small as a misshapen fire hose can have profound meaning when we learn to tap into intuition.

Creating Your Intuitive Soul Painting

- First, choose your medium, whether that is colored pencil, marker, pastel, colored pens, paint, even crayon, whatever your personal preference. I make sure to have red, blue, yellow, green, orange, purple, and magenta, but I occasionally use brown and black as well. I have been a watercolor artist for many years, so that is my medium of choice. I like the way that the colors can "accidentally" flow into each other, creating other colors and moving into other parts of the page. I also like that I can create blurry effects and control how opaque the image is. I use heavy watercolor paper so that it stays flat when I am painting. Do not be concerned if you "have no artistic ability." You do not need any to be successful in this exercise.

- Before you begin your painting, it can be helpful to ask your intuition a question you would like more information about, such as, "Can you tell me more about my health?" This can lend your work more focus.

- Write your name at the top of the page and ask your intuition to show you a color to start with. After some practice, you can draw or paint whatever images come to you, but I would suggest starting with a human figure or something else, like a flower or plant, in the shape of a human figure, with human body parts. These are the easiest to interpret.

- As you begin, feel free to add whatever comes to you, including words, energy, and messages from the "other side." Try
  not to think; just listen and feel. The work will not be hung
  in a museum and it will not be judged. Whatever colors and
  shapes you feel drawn to, put them on the paper. My figures
  are seldom ever in anatomically correct proportion, and the
  colors do not usually correspond to the chakra where they
  are located. Don't worry about making the creation resemble
  you in any way; this is just a symbolic interpretation.

- Continue working on your drawing or painting until you
  intuitively feel it is finished. This may take you only a few
  minutes or a much longer time. Enjoy the process and follow
  wherever it leads you.

Interpreting Your Painting

Interpreting these paintings for yourself starts with asking
what the overall image means to you or what it might remind
you of. Then you can refer to a color symbolism chart of your
choice, which you can find online, or you can use mine found
on the following page.

Next, consider which parts of the painting you created first.
The meanings of those colors usually reflect the first impres-
sion of how you view yourself, or perhaps what you most need
to learn.

Work your way down the page, paying attention to the
placement of the colors, shapes, sizes of body parts (especially
if they are irregular), whether or not you made a neck on your
image or if that area is absent (meaning communication may
be difficult), and if you are missing any body parts. I'd recommend referring to a book, such as *You Can Heal Your Life* by
Louise Hay, to look up the symbolic meaning of body parts.
You can also search the internet for this information. For example, legs and feet are associated with moving forward in

Color	Symbolism
Red	Anger, energy, love/hate, stop, attention, power, blood
Blue	Empathic abilities, calm, likes water, sensitive, trust, loyalty, sadness/depression, sky
Yellow	Intuition, joy, generosity, spiritual teacher, sun, warmth, happiness, jealousy
Green	Growth, new life, spring, nature, renewal, money, greed
Purple	Intuition, spirituality, psychic ability, religion, wisdom, dignity
Orange	Adventure, courage, energy, creativity, determination, sexuality, enthusiasm, individuality, intelligence
Magenta	Own style, unique, not afraid to be different, dramatic, harmonious, creative, bold
Pink	Hope, blend of high energy and calm, childlike, creative, sweet, playful, feminine

life. If your image doesn't have them, you may feel stuck, or if they're pointing in two different directions, you may have choices to make or feel conflicted.

Pay attention to symbols and other images. Search the internet for the various meanings of what you've painted, such as diamonds, squares, animals, etc. There are often multiple meanings associated with a given symbol, so use the meaning that most resonates with you. Listen to messages from your intuition as you scan the painting, and it will help you interpret your work. Be open and don't judge, even if what you hear from your intuition seems "weird" or may not make sense. Just go with it. It will make sense later.

I *strongly* recommend creating an Intuitive Soul Painting for yourself as you work through the chapters of this book and identify your individual issues and strengths. Create more paintings at various stages of your healing process so you can see your progress and growth.

TECHNIQUE THREE: DREAM INTERPRETATION

Dream Interpretation, Jungian-Style

Dreaming is another way we receive information from our intuition and our bodies as well as from loved ones who have passed. When we are awake, we can push down our feelings and trauma, but sleep ignites our unconscious minds and connections to the "other side," helping us let go of numbing fear. Dreaming is a way of getting our attention and bringing issues and emotions to the surface so we can process them. The best way to stop nightmares from reoccurring is to process and interpret them, since the themes and messages are often a compilation of fear accumulated over many years, but our inclination is to try to block them out and forget them.

Dreams are also an important medium for people who have passed to spend time with us and give us messages. When you dream about people who have died and it feels like they are really there with you, they are. Those are some of my favorite dreams.

How to interpret your dreams, using Jungian psychology:

- Write down every detail you can remember about your dream as soon as you wake up. Colors you saw, the way you felt, if the scenes were familiar or if they reminded you of somewhere, the people, everything—don't leave anything out.

- Ask yourself if you received an overall message or meaning or if there was an overall theme. There is no right or wrong answer, just what it meant to you.

- Next, dissect each object, person, scene, color, and symbol. Ask yourself what they mean to you, how they made you feel, and look up the various possible meanings for the symbols and objects where appropriate. Don't feel restricted to the common symbolic meaning of any particular object. Your dream was meant specifically for you. For example, if you dream about an elephant, ask yourself what elephants make you think of, then look up any symbolic meanings and write down whatever resonates with you.

- Once you have determined, to the best of your ability, the meanings of the individual parts of your dream, see if you can fit them together into a theme or a general lesson. Perhaps there will be more than one. Again, there is no right or wrong answer, just what the dream means to you. If your intuition needs to tell you the message again, you will have the dream or a similar one again. If you have nightmares, make sure you take the time to discern their meanings. They are delivering important messages.

TECHNIQUE FOUR: ORACLE CARDS, PENDULUMS, AND RUNES

There are various tools I use to help me "talk" with my intuition. I often ask a question and let my pendulum spin, draw an oracle or angel card, or choose one or two rune stones to guide me. Have fun and experiment with different methods. Some may resonate with your intuition and others may not, so do whatever works best for you.

Oracle Cards

I begin my readings by consulting an oracle card deck. This helps me clear my head, begin connecting with my intuition and guides, and start focusing on the client's issues.

You can use oracle cards to guide you with specific questions, to start your day, or to receive general information from your intuition. When I searched the internet for oracle cards, I found over five thousand different options with themes like angels, animals, mythological creatures, fairies, the moon, and the Virgin Mary, just to name a few. Some people use tarot cards rather than oracle cards.

To select a card, I spread them out in my hand and close my eyes. I touch the cards until I "feel" one that I am guided to. You can also spread the cards out on the floor or a table and choose one or shuffle and randomly choose from the pile. There is no wrong way to do this. I just choose one card, but you can choose multiple cards for more information or to clarify the message from other cards.

Most decks have an accompanying book that contains detailed descriptions of the cards, but not always their meanings. You will need to determine the meaning intuitively and decide which parts of the card or cards resonate with you and which that don't. Often these books give suggestions for various ways to draw the cards, interpret them, and use them for guidance.

Pendulums

There are multiple techniques for using pendulums. Some people "douse" over oracle cards, meaning that they slowly move the pendulum over the spread-out deck until the pendulum begins to spin. Others use the pendulum in the same way over the body when doing energy healings to see what parts of the body need special attention. I tend to use mine for yes-or-no questions and for asking about whether or not supplements, food, and occasional medications and doses are appropriate. Start with this technique and then explore different options!

- Decide how "yes" and "no" will be indicated. I have directed my pendulum to spin clockwise for "yes" and counterclockwise for "no."
- Wrap the chain around your first two fingers and place them on your forehead with the pendulum hanging down. You will be looking down at the pendulum with your head tilted forward.

- Begin with the pendulum still and then ask your question.
- You'll be amazed that every time it starts spinning. In between questions, it often stops on its own before spinning again.

Runes

Runes are stones used originally by the Vikings. They come in a set of twenty-four with an ancient symbol on each, usually with a book to help with interpretation of the message or messages you receive. You can ask a particular question before drawing a rune or runes, or simply ask for information to help guide you through the day. You can spread them out facedown on a table or make your choice from the bag they often come in, using your intuition as a guide to pick those that call to you.

You can also connect to intuition through meditation, yoga, energy healing, acupuncture, exercise, grounding, and more. There is no right or wrong way to connect with your intuition. We all experience this connection differently so feel free to explore and never judge others.

END OF CHAPTER 5 QUESTIONS

1. What questions can you ask your intuition? What did you find easy and difficult about that process?
2. How do you receive intuitive information? Words, images, physical touch, feelings, smells?
3. Which tools for connecting to your intuition do you think you will try first?
4. How did you feel when creating your Intuitive Soul Painting? What did you learn?
5. What is your favorite way of connecting to intuition and why? What way do you feel is most accurate?

6. Could you relate to the information about childhood intuitive and psychic abilities? What were yours? Did you have anyone you could share them with?

7. What do you think are your blocks to connecting with intuition? How can you overcome them?

Symptoms Are Signals from Our Intuition

It is by going down into the abyss that we recover the
treasures of life. Where you stumble, there lies your
treasure.

—Joseph Campbell

Carl Jung was one of the first to write and talk about working
with symptoms and conditions as signals from our intuition.
This does not mean that your physical and emotional symptoms are not real or that you have somehow caused them. Nor
does it mean that physical root causes and contributors to illness are less valid than emotional or spiritual ones.

However, the concept of symptoms as messages from our
intuition does help explain why certain parts of the body or
issues are impacted, often repeatedly. For example, empathic
people who feel their own emotions in their guts, as well as other
people's, often develop digestive symptoms, irritable bowel syndrome, and constipation or diarrhea. Very sensitive people,
individuals who constantly worry about others or those who
spend more time and energy caring for others than themselves,
commonly develop symptoms in the 4th chakra—the heart or
the breasts. People with unresolved anger often develop liver-
related symptoms. My signal for when I am not being present

and not listening to my intuition enough is weight gain. Symbolically, weight can be about grounding, since heavier things are pulled to the earth using gravity more intensely than lighter objects. Grounding helps us be more present. These are all instances in which a habitual physical symptom has an equally real emotional or spiritual connection.

The concept of symptoms being signals from our intuition goes deeper than just explaining why we develop illness. Listening to our intuition helps us to live authentically and find our life path(s), while trauma, illness, unhappiness, or accidents distract us. If we are allowing fear to prevent us from expressing our feelings, leave unhappy relationships, or start our dream business, we are also allowing that fear to prevent us from being our true selves. Our intuition wants us to live full, happy lives, without anything in our way. I believe that this is why we are all here, the ultimate life purpose, if you will: to be our authentic selves, whatever that may mean. When we stray from that path, our intuition, using our bodies and emotions, has to get our attention.

I strongly believe in the power of this approach, and it was instrumental in my healing from both bulimia and Lyme disease. I will discuss more of my experience with Lyme disease in part 2, but when I dialogued with the Lyme disease and my intuition, I received the message that I was afraid of moving forward with my life. I was afraid of being vulnerable, being exposed, and also of success. It was time to stop avoiding writing my book, which I had first been told about by my guides when I was sixteen. I knew that if I wanted to recover, I needed to start taking the first steps and eventually finish the book proposal.

Since Lyme disease is a potentially life-threatening condition that impacts the entire body, it would be classified under the 7th chakra, along with other chakras, depending on the other parts of the body impacted. The message I received during the dialogue was also appropriate to the 7th chakra because it was about life purpose, being authentic, and connecting with Spirit. Bulimia, which is a 3rd chakra illness because it deals with addiction and body image, and the 5th chakra because the throat and teeth are impacted by vomiting, was symbolic of expressing feelings, needing to learn to love and accept myself and my body, needing to express my authenticity, which are also 3rd and 5th chakra issues. There is a reason why we develop certain issues and illnesses and where they occur. There are no accidents. As I stated before, the longer we ignore these symptoms, or signals from our bodies and intuition, the more intense they have to become to get our attention. The key is to listen and respond early, no matter how frightening it can be.

Louise Hay wrote what has become a classic guidebook about the symbolism and meaning of the parts of the body and related illness. *You Can Heal Your Life* is a great tool, along with this book, for learning more about some of the possible root causes and contributors for the issues you have encountered. I also love traditional Chinese medicine (TCM) for learning more about symbolism and the body.

The fundamental concepts of TCM are harmony, or the balance of yin and yang (opposing forces or opposites), and the flow of energy in and around the body, called qi. If one system or body part is out of balance, it throws off the harmony of the entire body and disrupts qi. Another name for qi is "life force." Different organs and parts have different properties based on characteristics of the seasons and certain elements, such as heat, moisture, fire, and air. I cannot begin to explain all of the intricacies of TCM here, but I encourage you to read more about this fascinating, ancient practice and consult with TCM practitioners.

In the following chapters, you will be learning even more about the symbolism of symptoms and parts of the body using the chakras. I strongly urge you to continue to ask yourself how your specific symptoms relate to the physical, emotional, and spiritual events you have experienced, your emotional characteristics, your beliefs, and what living authentically means to you.

7

Identifying Individual Issues and Strengths

We cannot change anything unless we accept it.
Condemnation does not liberate, it oppresses.

—Carl Jung

It would be helpful to have paper and pen ready for this chapter. You will be learning a great deal about yourself and identifying the issues you need and want to work on as well as your strengths.

My clients often come to me after having negative experiences with the traditional medical system. I've learned that doctors primarily treat symptoms rather than try to discover the root issue, leading to patients who stay sick and/or who are dissatisfied with their care.

Part of the reason for this is that ten or fifteen minutes is all the time that insurance companies and Medicare will allow. In many cases, the predetermined fees barely pay for salaries, overhead, mortgages, student loans, and other expenses. You can't blame some medical professionals for refusing to even participate with insurance.

This short period of time is hardly enough to explore when the issues started, the severity of the symptoms, or to explain how essential details like sleep, stress, exercise, and diet will impact your health. It is faster and easier just to prescribe a pill, tell people to lose weight, or order expensive, often inconclusive tests. If we're lucky, we actually get an explanation of what our test results mean, but usually we're just handed a set of numbers. Or more often, we are just told that everything is normal, even though we still feel unhealthy.

I have heard far too many stories of patients who were not taken seriously when they told their doctors that they were sick. They were ignored when they asked for more in-depth testing and ridiculed when they asked about things like Lyme disease, Hashimoto's thyroiditis, vaccine reactions, rare diseases, autoimmune disease, or vitamin deficiencies. Far too often they were told that their issues were psychological and psychiatric medications were prescribed. They later learned that their conditions were physical, not emotional, but it often took years to get a proper diagnosis.

I believe that we need to take a different approach, which I call "patient-based root cause medicine." This approach puts the patients' needs first, rather than insurance company profits. It works by actually listening to patients and figuring out what is truly happening and devoting sufficient time and energy to addressing all possible causes, whether they be physical, emotional, or spiritual.

Most people are familiar with the relationship between stress and physical and even emotional symptoms. Stress has been shown to lower the immune response, interfere with sleep, and produce cortisol, which, according to research published on Mayoclinic.org, disrupts the reproductive system and growth process. Long-term stress puts you at risk of many health problems, including anxiety, depression, digestive problems, headaches, heart disease, weight gain, and memory and concentration impairment.

When I talk about emotional and spiritual root causes, I

am talking about much more specific things than just stress in general. I want to know when the stress started and what caused it. What were the circumstances? What are your family dynamics and family history? What early trauma and feelings might you have pushed down? Have you been able to be your true self or have you hidden yourself, fearing rejection and abandonment?

If we do not identify specific issues, we cannot address them. The chakra chart included on page 67 is at the heart of my work with clients. I describe where the seven chakras are located and which parts of the body and what organs correspond with them. I also include the related emotional and spiritual issues and descriptions.

As you will see when you answer the questions about your own health and wellness, our issues don't fit into neat little boxes. Many conditions as well as organs, glands, and body parts correspond to more than one chakra. Creative blocks are a great example. Stalled creativity may result from blockage in the 2nd or 5th chakra. The 2nd chakra involves the reproductive organs, the hips, and lower back and concerns creativity, relationships, career, and money. The 5th chakra is in the throat area and has to do with expression.

Creativity in any form is highly personal and can be terrifying because you risk exposing your innermost feelings. You put yourself out there for the world to see and risk rejection, ridicule, failure, and, for perfectionists, never being happy with the outcome.

If you were told by your family that being an artist or expressing yourself was shameful or that you would fail, that brings the 1st chakra into the mix, which concerns safety, security, family, and belonging. Physically, it corresponds to your bones, immune system, blood, and extremities. Depending on your situation, other chakras could be impacted as well.

DIRECTIONS FOR THIS CHAPTER

You are going to be creating your own chakra report, about your unique situation, from information you hear from yourself and your intuition, just like I do for a client. The report will identify different symptoms and issues and associate them with one or more chakras. As you learn about each of the chakras in the following chapters, you will refer to this report to help you identify the various methods of healing that may be right for you.

Using the checklist that follows, ask yourself these questions to help determine where you may have issues based on the chakras. Take note of which questions you answer yes or no to and the chakras that correspond with them. Take your time and write down what issue came to mind as you read each question, relevant background information, and anything else you feel is important. As always, allow yourself to be guided by intuition. You will later input this information into your personal chakra report.

More than one chakra may be listed after certain questions because the physical symptoms and emotions relate to more than one part of the body. For example, the second group of questions relates to messages we may have received from family or others (chakras 1 and 2), self-esteem (chakra 3), picking up feelings empathically from others (chakra 6), and difficulties expressing yourself (chakra 5).

PERSONAL CHAKRA ISSUE CHECKLIST

- Do you find yourself having self-deprecating or self-critical thoughts? Do you criticize your body, your abilities, your choices, your appearance, etc.? Are you judgmental toward yourself, and do you tell yourself that you aren't capable of doing things before you have even tried? Chakras 3, 2.

- Are you fearful? Are there things you want to do that you have never even tried because you have been told you can't, or because you have told yourself you can't? What are they? Are you afraid of what people will say about you? Chakras 1, 2, 3, 5, 6.

- Do you know what you want, and are you able to express how you feel? Do you know what is important to you? Chakras 5, 7.

- Do you trust and communicate with your intuition, or do you have to be in control? Chakras 6, 7.

- Are you a helicopter parent, or do you let your children have their independence? Chakras 1, 2, 4.

- Are you able to live in the moment and be mindful, or are you always thinking about the past or the future? Chakras 1, 6, 7.

- Do you have any guilt or grief? Chakras 4, 1.

- Are you always thinking about what you eat, what you weigh, and how you look? Do you have a realistic idea of your body shape, or do you have body dysmorphia? Chakras 3, 6.

- Do you have any food sensitivities? Do you have issues with your gut? Do you have gut symptoms when nervous or upset? Chakra 3.

- What supplements do you take and why? All chakras.

- Does your career make you happy, or do you dream about doing something else? If you are not happy, what would you like to be doing? Chakra 2.

- Are you able to relax and be alone with your thoughts, or are you distracted and uncomfortable? Chakras 6, 1.

- Are you burdened by grief, depression, and/or anxiety? Chakras 1, 6, 3.

- Are you able to set appropriate boundaries, or are you codependent? Are you empathic? Do you pick up the energies of other people and become unable to let go of them? Chakras 4, 2, 6.

- If you have psychic or intuitive abilities, are you comfortable with them, or are you afraid of them? Chakras 6, 7.

- Do you have a chronic illness? Are you in pain or discomfort frequently? When did these issues start, and what have you tried to remedy them? Chakras 7, 1, and potentially others depending on the symptoms.

- Do you eat a diet as free of chemicals, GMOs, sugar, hormones, processed foods, and antibiotics as possible? Do you eat enough vegetables and get enough vitamins, minerals, proteins, and fats? What foods don't agree with you? Chakras 3, 6, 1.

- Do you filter your water? Chakras 6, 3.

- Can you be true to yourself? Are you authentic? If not, why do you think that is? Chakras 1, 3, and 5.

- Are you sensitive to chemicals, medications, strong scents, or mold? Do you avoid chemicals, artificial fragrances, plastics, xenoestrogens, and electromagnetic fields? Do you find yourself using prescription or over-the-counter medications on a daily or regular basis? Chakras 6, 3, potentially others.

- Do you avoid situations that will cause stress and regularly release stress through relaxation, recreational activities, meditation, exercise, and more? Chakras 2, 6, 3.

- Do you detoxify your mind and body by taking breaks from social media, spending time alone, using saunas, coffee enemas, or exercise that makes you sweat? Chakras 2, 3, 7.

- Do you spend time with people you care about, and do you have a support network? Chakras 2, 1, 4.

- Do you have people you can talk to and share your intimate feelings with? Chakras 5, 4.

- Do you have a relationship with a higher power, God, your intuition, nature, or some spiritual power? Chakras 6, 7.
- Do you engage in creative activities? Chakra 2.
- Have you had any surgeries or serious injuries? All chakras.
- Any addiction issues? What about family or close friends? Chakra 3, 1, possibly 2.
- Are you fatigued, do you have trouble sleeping, or do you just not feel like yourself? Chakras 7, 1, 2, potentially others.
- Have you lost interest in sex and romantic relationships, or are you having sexual dysfunction? Chakras 2, 4, 3.
- Are you dealing with a dysfunctional family situation and letting it take up much of your time and your thoughts? Chakras 1, 6, 3.
- Are you dealing with emotional issues or mental illness? Have you in the past? Does mental illness run in your family? Chakras 6, 1.

This list of questions will not address every potential problem or strength, and I encourage you to use the chakra descriptions in the next step to pinpoint issues you have not identified by using the questionnaire. The issues you identify may be minor annoyances or more significant problems, and it's up to you to decide how or if you would like to address them. A good rule of thumb is if the issue is interfering with your quality of life, relationships, work, or your health, it may be prudent to work to address it. I have also identified strengths, abilities, and qualities I like about myself.

As an example, these would be some of the items on my list:

- Medications and supplements: Armour Thyroid, estrogen patch, testosterone cream, low dose of antidepressant, supplements for adrenals, anti-inflammatory, multivitamin with iron, omega-3, B-complex, hyaluronic acid, glucosamine and chondroitin.

- Very happy and fulfilled in my career. Have set goals for advancement and helping more people.

- Chronic issues and when they started: Ongoing shoulder pain and range-of-motion issues that started about a year ago while doing pole fitness, intermittent knee pain, gluten and dairy intolerance, generalized anxiety (much improved from the past), intermittent insomnia, hypothyroid.

- I eat as organically as possible and filter my water for fluoride, chlorine, chloramines, and more.

- Definitely true to myself. Have worked very hard to gain self-love, self-acceptance, and authenticity. Strengths and skills: determination, emotional and physical strength, creativity, strong spiritual beliefs, being sensitive and an empath (while these can also make life difficult).

- Sensitive to chemicals, mold, artificial scents.

- My preferred forms of stress reduction are creativity, writing, exercise six days a week, pole dancing, meditation.

- What makes me happy: Spending time with my husband, daughters, and their families; movement and pole dance; being at the beach or just outside; collecting sea glass; traveling; helping people heal and grow; being creative.

- I have a very strong support network—husband, daughters, friends. When I was growing up my support network was primarily maternal grandparents and friends.

- Very strong relationship with Spirit and my intuition.

- Surgery to remove uterus and one ovary. Rare carcinoid tumor.

- Family history: mental illness, gambling addiction, binge and emotional eating.

- Stressors and trauma: Growing up in a dysfunctional family, being bullied, my mother getting sick and the family situation that developed.
- What I would like to change: More patience, less self-doubt and perfectionism, better time management, body dysmorphia, sleep more consistently.
- Excellent at boundary setting; mindfulness isn't always easy; working on grounding more.

CREATING YOUR CHART

Now that you've created your own list based on the questions, read over the complete list of chakras and their descriptions to become familiar with them. As you read, make note of the chakras that resonate with you, even if you don't think your symptoms correspond with them. There is no such thing as an incorrect observation. Just listen to what you hear from your

Emotional	Physical
7TH CHAKRA	**7TH CHAKRA**
(Crown) Purpose in life, relationship with Spirit	Life-threatening illnesses, chronic illnesses, brain, nervous system, overview of the body and spirit
6TH CHAKRA	**6TH CHAKRA**
(Third eye) Intuition, psychic ability, ability to perceive and make judgments about the world, morality, flexibility, ability to change and fit into society without changing so much that you lose yourself, mood, mental illness	Headaches, including migraines; vision and hearing issues; sensitivity to mold, chemicals, scents, and other toxins; brain tumor; stroke; neurological diseases or injury

Emotional	Physical
5TH CHAKRA	**5TH CHAKRA**
(Throat) Self-expression—too much or not enough, will and determination, making things happen vs. waiting for things to happen, communication authenticity, activism, judgment and criticism	Thyroid issues, dental problems, teeth grinding, acid reflux, neck alignment or injury, rotator-cuff injuries, tonsillitis, chronic sore throat
4TH CHAKRA	**4TH CHAKRA**
(Heart) Expressing emotions—too much or not enough, love, intimacy, nurturing, grief, parenting—helicopter or neglect, giving vs. getting help, being an empath, sensitivity, self vs. others—boundaries, codependency	Heart disease, blood pressure, cancer of any of these areas, asthma, COPD, lungs, breasts, pneumonia, bronchitis
3RD CHAKRA	**3RD CHAKRA**
(Solar plexus) Eating disorders, body image, self-esteem—not enough or narcissism, responsibility to yourself vs. others, self-care, perfectionism, ability to take criticism, pride	Gut and bowel issues, bacterial imbalance, food intolerances, ulcers, liver disease, addiction, adrenals, weight concerns, diabetes
2ND CHAKRA	**2ND CHAKRA**
(Sacral) Feminine/masculine energy balance, abuse trauma, creativity, career and work vs. personal time, intimacy, sexuality, including sexual identity	Fertility, PMS, endometriosis, fibroids, polycystic ovary syndrome, urinary problems, hormone imbalance, menopause, sexual dysfunction, back pain

Emotional	Physical
1ST CHAKRA	**1ST CHAKRA**
(Root) Family issues and family history, trust, safety, basic needs, caretaking, support systems and belonging, healthy boundaries	Blood diseases; autoimmune disorders; immune deficiency; AIDS; bones, joints, and muscles; skin; general inflammation; varicose veins; sciatica

intuition and write it down, adding to the list you initially created. A blank version of this Chakra Chart Worksheet that you can copy and fill in yourself can be found on pages 291-292.

Now that you have a sense of what issues and symptoms you'd like to focus on, take a look at the following fictional case and practice categorizing the symptoms by the chakra they might be associated with. Compare what you wrote down to my findings. You may have identified chakras and issues I did not, and that is perfectly all right. I hope that Mary's case will help you think about possibilities you may not have considered in your own situation.

PRACTICE CASE STUDY

Mary, a fifty-two-year-old woman, is having symptoms of anxiety, insomnia, mild depression, fatigue, night sweats, occasional inflammation in her joints, and brain fog. She has become less tolerant of dairy and has gut issues that are inconsistent. She has not been able to receive a definitive diagnosis. She is also light-headed sometimes, and her blood pressure tends to run below normal.

She takes a good multivitamin, enjoys yoga and exercise but doesn't do it as much as she would like, and would like to lose about fifteen pounds. She was able to lose twenty pounds by increasing her exercise last year and hasn't gained it back. She craves sugar and carbohydrates. She is sensitive to strong fragrances.

She grew up in a home with an alcoholic father and a mother who tried but was pretty overwhelmed so didn't have time to devote to her daughter like Mary truly needed. Mary, at age twenty, married her boyfriend after becoming pregnant. She was happy to get out of the house but put off college. She has since gone on to earn her MBA and run her own company but is feeling unfulfilled.

She has always enjoyed flowers and gardening and recently took a class in floral design, which she loves. She recently divorced her husband after forty years, knowing she should have ended the marriage long ago. She hasn't been intimate with anyone for five years. She has a great relationship with her three children but is very concerned about her youngest daughter, whom she believes has become addicted to opioids after back pain from a car accident. Mary is hesitant to say anything to her because she doesn't want to upset her.

Her mother, whom she never had the easiest relationship with, passed away recently after a long illness, dementia. Her father passed away about ten years before. Mary also has a family history of heart disease, diabetes, glaucoma, and mental illness. Mary had been her mother's sole caregiver because her siblings lived too far away. It was an almost full-time job, and Mary had very little time for herself or for self-care. She feels guilty for being relieved that her mother has passed away, even though her mother was a very negative person and it deeply affected Mary's moods whenever she was with her, but she now knows that this negativity was about her mother and not about her.

Before reading my description of what chakras I would cite to categorize Mary's issues, give it a try yourself. Just categorize the information with the chakra you think is most appropriate. No interpretation is needed. Take a screenshot on your phone or print it out so it's in front of you when you go through the rest of the chapter. Warning: there are a lot of possible subtle nuances.

MY INTERPRETATION

What I would pay attention to first: Mary is female and fifty-two. She is likely menopausal or post-menopausal, so that would apply to the 2nd chakra. She is having some possible hormonal symptoms like anxiety, insomnia, fatigue, brain fog, and night sweats. These symptoms could also be explained by other things, like adrenal fatigue, stress, general anxiety, side effects to medication, and more.

7th Chakra

Overall, Mary's quality of life is not the way she would like it to be. She is unfulfilled and is unsure of her life purpose. She has been devoting her life to others. Many of her symptoms have been chronic, like fatigue, inflammation, and insomnia. She would benefit from a stronger relationship with Spirit and intuition. She is capable of exerting discipline, though, having lost twenty pounds and kept it off. She has a good amount of personal insight.

6th Chakra

The symptoms that fit into this chakra are anxiety, brain fog, sensitivity to strong fragrances, family history of glaucoma, and need for more connection to intuition and self. When she listens to her intuition and trusts it, she is always glad she did.

5th Chakra

The symptoms that fit into this chakra for Mary are difficulty speaking up and expressing her opinions and a tendency to push down her feelings, however, she has made great progress in this area, as evidenced by leaving her unhappy marriage.

4th Chakra

Mary is very empathic and easily picks up the moods of people around her, like she did with her mother. Boundaries are an issue. She hates the idea of possibly hurting the feelings of the people she cares about, like her family. At her job, she is able to be more direct and manage people without taking things personally. There is a family history of heart disease. Anxiety can also relate to the 4th chakra because of heart-rate changes. Mary is a natural caregiver, nurturing and kind.

3rd Chakra

The issues Mary has that fit into this chakra are gut issues, cravings, food intolerances, relationship between mood and gut symptoms, boundaries, blood sugar, light-headedness (adrenals), fatigue, self-esteem, self-care, and weight. As I have said, though, she was able to modify her behavior and diet and lose weight and keep it off.

2nd Chakra

Mary's 2nd chakra issues are hormones, menopause, career decisions, relationships, the need for stress relief, and more relaxation and exercise. Also, the need for intimacy, and body image. She is intelligent and resourceful, having received her MBA, and is now taking classes in things that spark joy.

1st Chakra

Dysfunctional family issues and trust, lack of security as a child, inflammation, family history of autoimmune disease (heart disease and diabetes), blood pressure, and not being able to be her authentic self.

As I have identified, Mary is dealing with quite a few issues and has areas of potential growth. She has work she can do in every energy center. I have found that this is the case with the vast majority of people I have worked with. You can also see that these energy centers and issues are not isolated or separate from each other. They are interconnected and impact each other directly.

Growing up in an alcoholic home impacted Mary's self-esteem and made her feel like she didn't deserve to have a voice. She got into a romantic relationship with someone who didn't appreciate her or listen to her, and she ended up having unprotected sex, getting pregnant, and feeling like she had to get married. She stayed with her husband, even though she was unhappy, because she didn't feel empowered until much later in life.

The stress of all of this led to many physical and emotional symptoms as well as entering into a career that has left her feeling unfulfilled. She was never taught how to listen to her intuition, or even that she had intuition. If she had, she would have been able to allow herself to embrace her creativity and likely would have taken a totally different path.

How'd it go for your assessment? What was your interpretation of Mary's symptoms? There is no right or wrong answer, but hopefully this exercise will help you to more easily identify and categorize your own issues according to the chakras.

Now that you've practiced connecting symptoms with various chakras, it's time to do the same with your own list of symptoms. Make a copy of the blank chakra report at the end of this book. Referring back to your list of symptoms and issues, place the items on your list where you think they fit on the chakra chart. Some items may be listed multiple times if they correspond to more than one chakra. For example, difficulty expressing your feelings could be listed under the

5th chakra, which deals with expression, but it can also apply to the 3rd chakra, which focuses on self-esteem. You may add to your list as you fill out the chart.

Here's an example of what my chart might look like based on the list of symptoms I shared.

Emotional		Physical	
7TH CHAKRA		**7TH CHAKRA**	
(Crown) Purpose in life, relationship with spirit	Purposes in life: helping people through my current work, spreading love and healing, raising children that will spread love and caring. I have a strong relationship with God/Spirit.	Life-threatening illnesses, chronic illnesses, brain, nervous system, overview of the body and spirit	No life-threatening illnesses. Have dealt with ongoing depression/anxiety in the past. Sleep can be challenging.
6TH CHAKRA		**6TH CHAKRA**	
(Third eye) Intuition, psychic ability, ability to perceive and make judgments about the world, morality, flexibility, ability to change and fit into society without changing so much that you lose yourself, mood, mental illness	I have a strong connection to my intuition, which I continue to develop. Psychic and medium abilities. Have learned to be more flexible and not such a control freak, but that is always a work in progress. ☺	Head, nose, ears, anxiety, etc.; pituitary gland; making and storing of hormones; pineal gland	Sensitivity to chemicals, artificial scents, mold. Live as non-toxically and organically as possible. Anxiety can be an issue, but as long as I process it, it isn't a problem. Sinus issues at times— allergies to grass, some animal furs. If I get headaches, they are usually sinus-related.

Emotional		Physical	
5TH CHAKRA		**5TH CHAKRA**	
(Throat) Self-expression—too much or not enough, will and determination, making things happen vs. waiting for things to happen, communication authenticity, activism, judgment and criticism	I am able to express my feelings and opinions appropriately. I can manifest what I want and work toward my goals, while also being open to letting go of control. Strong-willed. Good communicator.	Throat, mouth, teeth, thyroid, neck	Hold stress in neck and shoulders. Have worked on flexibility with chiropractor. Ongoing issue with right shoulder from pole dance. Teeth grinder, wear retainers at night from Invisalign treatment. Hypothyroid—use Armour Thyroid.
4TH CHAKRA		**4TH CHAKRA**	
(Heart) Emotions, nurturance, partnership, giving vs. getting help, care of others	Very empathic and sensitive. Nurturing and caring. Able to set appropriate boundaries, but that was learned. Tendency to do things for myself but better at asking for help. Work well with others.	Heart, lungs, blood pressure, cholesterol, breasts	No issues here. Used to have lower-than-normal blood pressure. Main stress relief is exercise—pole 6–8 hours a week and daily walking 2–3 miles.
3RD CHAKRA		**3RD CHAKRA**	
(Solar plexus) Eating disorders, body image, self-esteem—not enough or narcissism, responsibility to yourself vs. others, self-care, perfectionism, ability to take criticism, pride	Strong self-esteem, definitely had to be learned. Still tend to be hard on myself and perfectionistic, but try to use it constructively. Very determined and disciplined when I want to be. Take time for emotional, physical, and spiritual self-care, but always working on improving. History of eating disorder, still some body dysmorphia.	Small intestine, stomach, addictions, liver, adrenal, hormones, blood sugar, gallbladder, kidneys, spleen	Feel my emotions in my gut with symptoms of nausea, cramping, occasional diarrhea, but tend toward constipation. Some food intolerances, strongly avoid gluten and dairy. Used to have hypoadrenalism, use adrenal support. Need to pay attention to blood sugar as it gets low.

Emotional		Physical	
2ND CHAKRA		**2ND CHAKRA**	
(Sacral) Balancing, relationships vs. money, you and I vs. we, creativity	I am able to make time for my personal life as well as my work life. Excellent marriage with soulmate. Supportive friends, but tend to be a bit of a loner, introverted but enjoy others. Very creative, used to paint professionally. Just started to make a little time for that. Need more creative activities.	Reproductive organs, bladder, prostate, large intestine, lower back	Had uterus and one ovary removed. Carcinoid tumor removed from appendix. Use bioidentical hormones. Menopause complete at age 50. Actively work on opening hips and stretching hip flexors.
1ST CHAKRA		**1ST CHAKRA**	
(Root) Family issues and family history, trust, safety, basic needs, caretaking, support systems and belonging, healthy boundaries	Dysfunctional family background—mental illness including bipolar, borderline personality disorder, narcissism, depression, anxiety, gambling addiction. Wasn't able to express myself or be authentic. Trust, safety, security issues in the past. Was a caregiver for several years for ill mother. Have done a lot of work on these issues.	Base of spine, blood, joints, bones, immune system, lymph system, allergies, skin	Some degeneration in spine and upper neck from gymnastics injury and osteopenia, which has been reversed with exercise. Strong immune system, supplements including multivitamin, glucosamine and chondroitin, omega-3, curcumin. Skin can be sensitive, occasional psoriasis on scalp. Some joint inflammation from exercise. Ferritin (iron stores) tends to run low.

Now that you've created your own chakra report, it's time to learn more about the chakras themselves. Chapters 8–14 in this book explore chakras 7 to 1. I recommend reading chapter 8 about the 7th chakra first, since it is an overview of the body. It will be helpful to read about all of the chakras in the following chapters, since if one isn't functioning properly, it will impact your entire being. However, if you wish, you can start with the chakra chapters that you most identify your symptoms with.

At this point, I recommend creating a symbolic painting for yourself such as the one described in chapter 5, if you haven't already. It is not a requirement but it will give you additional information about your issues.

As you read, you will be recording a great deal of information about yourself, in a way you likely never have before. It may feel overwhelming and bring up feelings you have long ago pushed aside. Just allow the process, without judgment, and proceed as slowly as you need to. I would encourage you to seek assistance from a therapist if this information is difficult and traumatic to recall.

With the help of your intuition, pick *one* exercise, life change, or challenge you would like to tackle first and start there. The tools and suggestions in the following chapters will guide you in how to address the issues you have identified. I have successfully used these tools myself and to help others, so I know that they work.

Start small. Accomplishing just one goal will feel amazing and show you that you do not need to be afraid. Often, we can't even get started because the task at hand seems overwhelming. We set ourselves up to fail before we even try. Pick something that isn't too difficult, so you can accomplish it fairly quickly and build up your confidence.

Take note of which issues you think you can take care of yourself and which you need help with. Don't try to do everything yourself. You don't receive a badge of honor for pretending that you are in control at all times. It's a sign of strength to be able to admit that we don't have all of the answers and to relinquish some control to a higher power and caring people.

Please be patient with yourself and don't expect to heal or

change overnight. Change can be difficult and scary, especially
if it is related to trauma. It is important to remember that if you
have suffered from acute illness, trauma, or abuse, you have
developed strength, determination, and courage. It's common
to sometimes move three steps forward and one or even two
steps back. Even so, you are still ultimately moving forward.
I certainly experienced this during my healing and recoveries,
whether they were emotional, physical, or spiritual.

You're embarking on a beautiful journey of healing guided
by intuition. It's taken strength and courage to even open this
book and begin the work of looking deeply into your life. I
know that with patience, trust, and the guiding voice of your
intuition you will find healing and happiness.

REFLECTIONS ON CHAPTER 7

- Keep your notes and questionnaire answers so you can compare them over time and assess your progress. Seeing even
  one issue checked off can help you feel more confident and
  motivated.

- How did you feel when creating your personal list? Did you
  feel inspired or overwhelmed? Is there a small issue you can
  begin to address to help you feel more confident?

- Allow your intuition to answer the questions and give you
  information without judgment. As I described in the previous chapter, intuition comes from a place of self-love and
  self-acceptance. There are no right or wrong answers. Intuition is not there to condemn you or blame you for being
  sick or having issues.

- Try not to worry about how many issues you might have to
  address. This is not a contest. You are not flawed or dam-
  aged. This exercise is to help you assess and work toward
  solving problems and living a better life, not to create more
  anxiety.

- Make note of any dreams you have during this time. They can help you identify where you might need to prioritize or issues you have that you may not have considered. Remember that dreaming is another way our intuition and our bodies speak to us.

- Using the tools in the previous chapter, write to your body and body parts, just like I taught you to write to your intuition and your guides, to help you identify and get more information about issues.

- Ask trusted loved ones and friends to help you fill out the questionnaire checklist earlier in the chapter if you are wondering about issues you might want or need to address. Sometimes we are too close to ourselves to be objective.

CALL TO ACTION ITEMS RELATED TO EVERY CHAKRA

CALL TO ACTION

The "Call to Action" items found in chapters 8 through 14 are general suggestions that will help with any condition related to that specific chakra. They are steps you can take to work on overall physical, emotional, and spiritual health and wellness. Many of these practices can benefit all of the chakras, so I've listed these universally helpful practices here. These are good principles to keep in mind as you continue reading through each of the chakra chapters, and I'll touch on these themes in more detail later on.

Physical

1. Pay attention to how the parts of your body are connected, and don't ignore even "small" symptoms. High blood pressure and cholesterol aren't just about your heart, and diabetes isn't just about blood sugar. Taking medication to control symptoms isn't enough. Not only do we need to pay attention to our overall health, but often if we make improvements

in diet, exercise, stress reduction, or other areas, we may not require medication at all. There is no such thing as a minor symptom; they are all signals that we need to pay attention. If we listen when our bodies tell us to rest, we can probably keep from catching a full-blown cold, having an accident because we aren't paying attention, or even worse.

2. Seek to learn all root causes of your symptoms—physical, emotional, and spiritual. Temporary fixes and only treating physical issues is not enough.

3. Take actions that positively impact your well-being in general, such as creative and fun activities, exploring and learning more about subjects you are interested in, challenging yourself physically and intellectually, and developing a spiritual connection. These are all part of self-care.

4. Get an adequate amount of rest and sleep. Seven or eight hours is generally the rule for prime functioning, but you may need more or less. Listen to your body and pay attention to how you feel. Rest can take many forms and may include sleep, but we all need downtime to clear our heads and rejuvenate.

5. Eat a healthy diet with as few chemicals and hormones as possible. Avoid sugar and inflammatory foods like gluten and dairy. Eat mostly vegetables and fruits, balanced with complete proteins.

6. Remove as many toxins as possible from other areas of your life. Common sources of toxins include cleaning products, personal products, and decor, such as carpets. Go through your cleaning supplies and bathroom cabinets and replace as many things as you can with natural alternatives.

Emotional and Spiritual

1. Connect to a force more powerful than yourself. You may call it God, the universe, nature, Mother Earth, even intuition. We are not alone and we don't always have all the answers.

2. Allow yourself to feel emotions, even if they are difficult. We often push them down because we think they will be too painful or because we are afraid of what we might do as a result, such as confronting someone we are angry with when we have worked hard to "keep peace." Negative emotions that we push down just become more powerful, and when we ignore the negative, we also risk ignoring positive emotions.

3. Do not allow yourself to be defined by illness, trauma, or experiences. You are not a label. People *have* cancer, they *aren't* cancer. People are abused, they aren't abuse, and someone may have anxiety but that isn't who they are. It is easy to get caught up in the fear and stigma of illness or trauma, but that is just a small component of our lives. We are so much more than that.

8

The Complete Person

Healing Using the 7th Chakra

Man's task is . . . to become conscious of the contents that
press upward from the unconscious.

—Carl Jung

Overall themes: the whole,
we are all connected, spirituality

7TH CHAKRA

I begin my readings and reports with the 7th chakra. It's
found at the crown, or top of the head. The corresponding
color is white, since it is a combination of all of the colors,
or deep violet; either color is correct. Another name for this
chakra is the *Sahasrara,* meaning the "lotus of a thousand
petals."

This chakra is connected to our higher consciousness,
Spirit, God, and the rest of the universe. It relates to enlight-
enment, to connection to our own bodies and with each
other.

The 7th chakra is an overview of our physical, emotional,
and spiritual makeup. When I check in with this chakra,

Location	Physical Issues	Emotional and Spiritual Concerns
Top of head Pineal gland	Life-threatening and chronic illness Brain and nervous system Whole body issues Chronic fatigue not linked to a physical issue	Spiritual crisis, spirituality Serious mental illness Life Purpose Relationship with Spirit, faith Addiction

I get a feel for whether a person is generally healthy and what he or she is looking for guidance on. I receive information about chronic diseases that impact the entire body, overall mood, and issues that affect all of a person's life, like grief, a desire for purpose, connection to faith or Spirit, and more.

POSSIBLE PHYSICAL, EMOTIONAL, AND SPIRITUAL ROOT CAUSES FOR ISSUES IN THIS CHAKRA

- Lack of connection to Spirit and intuition
- Substance abuse
- Family dysfunction
- Trauma history
- Disconnection from the body
- Mental health issues
- Spiritual crisis

INTUITIVE WRITING PROMPTS

To begin a dialogue with your intuition that focuses on this chakra, you might ask:

- What can I do to feel more meaning in my life?
- What are some of my life purposes?
- How/what have I learned from adversity?

CALL TO ACTION

These are general suggestions that will help with any condition related to the 7th chakra. If you are having symptoms in this chakra, I believe that your intuition and Spirit are calling on you to work on the following if you want to attain physical, emotional, and spiritual health.

PHYSICAL

1. Make a list of any serious or life-threatening illnesses you have currently or have had in the past.
2. Notice any patterns, like issues with the same part of the body more than once. Often we will have recurring illnesses or injuries related to areas where we are most vulnerable.

EMOTIONAL AND SPIRITUAL

1. Think about the importance of faith in your life as well as spirituality and/or religious beliefs. Have there been times when your faith and spiritual life was stronger? How did that feel. Think about what goals you have for this area of your life.
2. Identify emotions and feelings that occur repeatedly. Any themes? How you would like to feel if you could?
3. Do not allow yourself to be defined by illness, trauma, or experiences. You are not a label.
4. Identify fears and other feelings related to death, and a belief or lack of belief in the afterlife.

AFFIRMATIONS AND VISUALIZATIONS FOR THE 7TH CHAKRA

Affirmations: Use and write these down. Carry them with you, put them in places you'll see them, or practice saying them to yourself throughout the day.

- I am safe.
- I am loved.
- I do not need to be in control.
- I can let go.

Visualizations:

- Visualize a warm protective light around your entire body. Allow it to envelope you, radiating from your 7th chakra at the crown of your head, down around your shoulders, and all the way to your feet. Allow yourself to feel whole, protected, and content.
- Practice grounding using the techniques mentioned in chapter 9.
- Practice mindfulness meditation.

CONDITION SPOTLIGHT

SPIRITUAL CRISIS AND SPIRITUAL AWAKENING

An important focus of the 7th chakra is the impact of spirituality and intuition on the mind, body, and soul. Our intuition is constantly talking with us and giving us messages about what we need, who is safe, decisions that are best for us, and more. If we are taught to listen, we can choose to respond or ignore it.

A spiritual crisis or awakening is related to intense "spiritual or intuitive events" and can occur when someone has difficulty coping with such an event, such as suddenly experiencing or discovering psychic or intuitive abilities, intense emotions, visions, remembering trauma, or experiencing a profound questioning of life or life purpose. The symptoms that can accompany spiritual crisis can be frightening and confusing and are often misdiagnosed as physical and mental illness. The terms "spiritual crisis" and "spiritual emergency" are often used interchangeably. Typical symptoms of spiritual emergency can include the following:

· Unusual or increased empathic, psychic, or similar spiritual experiences
· Feeling overwhelmed by responsibilities and activities of daily life
· Feeling very ungrounded and finding it difficult to be in the present
· Strong energy and tingling in various areas of the body
· Strong emotions and emotional fluctuations
· Feeling different from other people, more in tune with the paranormal and nature
· Intense anxiety and dread

To learn more about this subject, I highly recommend the books *Spiritual Emergency: When Personal Transformation Becomes A Crisis* by Stanislav and Christina Grof and *In Case of Spiritual Emergency* by Catherine G. Lucas.

A spiritual awakening can occur in conjunction with or separately from a spiritual crisis.

Lucas defines spiritual awakening as "above all a process; a process of exploration and unfolding, a process of learning and growth, of healing and purification. It involves the whole of our beings and works on all levels, physical, emotional and psychological, as well as spiritual." The intensity of this process determines whether it becomes a spiritual emergency, and different people will have profoundly different experiences.

How do you know if you are experiencing a spiritual awakening or spiritual emergency versus "just" having a physical or emotional health issue? It is my belief that every physical or emotional health issue can potentially be a spiritual awakening, if you avail yourself of the possibility.

If we are open to opportunities to awaken to Spirit and our intuition—whether that means learning from people we meet, changing negative or destructive habits, standing up for ourselves, or facing our fears—then we don't have to be smashed over the head with a sledgehammer by a spiritual crisis or emergency. If we ignore those inner voices and overwork ourselves, spend too much time on things that aren't really important, don't feed our souls, let fear control us, etc., then it takes something more serious to get our attention and force spiritual change.

If you consider mental or physical illness from a spiritual awakening or crisis point of view, it may explain why traditional approaches and treatments are not always effective. Perhaps the reason that diagnosed bipolar disorder, anxiety, and depression are often not helped by pharmaceuticals is because the real problem is spiritual, not chemical. What if we are medicating people when we should be helping them connect to their intuition and to love and accept themselves? One of the reasons why twelve-step programs have been so effective in helping addicts is because they are spiritual and help people give control to a higher power and transform their lives. The addiction itself might be a necessary process for some people to begin the spiritual transformation.

What can you do if you are going through a spiritual crisis? Here are some helpful suggestions:

- Do not be afraid to ask for help, but seek out professionals who are open to the concept of spiritual crisis and spirituality as it relates to the mind and body. Find a Jungian therapist or a person trained in spiritual crisis or emergency.

- You want support from people who are going to validate you, enhance, and listen to your intuition and not just band-aid your symptoms with medication. Seek out a professional who will search for every type of root cause and who understands that physical and emotional illness includes a spiritual component. Choose your practitioners carefully and remember that they are working *for* you. You can fire them if you aren't happy.

- Investigate mindfulness. Mindfulness means being present and aware of this day, this moment, and yourself. It gets your head out of the clouds and out of the confusion and chaos. There are wonderful books and CDs on mindfulness (see the resources in the appendix at the end of the book for recommendations). Many hospitals have mindfulness training programs. Being with your thoughts and feelings may not be comfortable, but trying to escape them won't make them go away.

- Try Kundalini yoga and meditation. Kundalini yoga helps you connect with your personal power and listen closely to your intuition and your body. Each lesson, or *kriya,* has a specific focus, such as a certain chakra or emotional state.

- Use the technique of Written Dialogue (see chapter 5) between yourself and your intuition. Keep a journal and do some simple art therapy. If you listen, you do not need the symptoms to get your attention in a negative way. Ask yourself what is important to you and what you need to be happy. This is a time to be following your dreams.

- Make a list of your fears and really be honest with yourself about why they exist. Are they left over from your childhood? Are they imposed by others? What will happen if you do something you are afraid of? Play that scenario out in your head. What is the worst thing that will happen if you take a chance? You have likely survived much worse. Are you holding yourself back because of fear of success or fear of failure?

- Take a look at the positive and negative in your life, including the people. If anything or anyone is holding you back, think about why you have kept them around. Be honest about the effects they are having on you.

Story: *The Red Book* and Jung's Spiritual Crisis

The Red Book is a famous work created by Carl Jung in 1913. It is also the result of a spiritual crisis. This book and the account of why and how it was written has provided great inspiration to me and is an excellent illustration of a spiritual emergency. The story of *The Red Book,* which concerns spiritual crisis and the 7th chakra, also connects to the 6th chakra with mental health, intuitive, and psychic experiences; the 4th chakra, which covers emotions; and the 2nd chakra, as applied to creativity. It's a great example of how interconnected all aspects of our health truly are.

During a very stressful time in his professional and personal life, Carl Jung began having uncontrollable visions of Europe flooded in blood. He went from having a tremendously successful career, material success, and a family, to being, as he describes it, immersed in chaos and torment.

He was constantly seeing images and felt that the visions were taking over. They were impacting his work as well as his private life and relationships. In an attempt to gain control over his life again, he began recording what he saw and heard in his head in the form of words and images. In order to do this, he allowed himself to go into waking trances and also communicated directly with spiritual guides and his intuition, which he felt were helping him and giving him messages. Eventually everything he had written and drawn was combined into one red leather-bound book.

The book was not published before Jung's death in 1961, and his heirs actually locked it into a vault, believing that it would discredit him. Finally, after repeated requests and fears that the book would fall into the hands of people who were Jung detractors, it was published in 2009. Despite the book being twelve by fifteen inches and weighing over ten pounds, more than fifty thousand copies have been sold. Ideas, theories, and techniques Jung learned from his work on *The Red Book* have influenced millions of people and continue to shape the world of psychology, self-help, and wellness today.

Many scholars have labeled what Jung experienced as a mental breakdown, but many others, myself included, call it a spiritual crisis. Not only was Jung learning to communicate with his intuition and receiving spiritual knowledge that would change the world, he was also receiving psychic information, which many Jung scholars believe were premonitions of World War I.

In writing *The Red Book,* Jung demonstrated extreme courage by challenging his own fears of what he thought was psychosis or even schizophrenia. Rather than listening to his colleagues and checking himself into a mental institution for treatment, he trusted his intuition and learned to communicate with it through waking trances and meditations. His story challenges the stigma of mental illness as something people should be ashamed of or that must be masked with psychotic medication.

By pushing down your feelings, visions, and intuition, you are potentially robbing yourself of valuable information that can help you heal and enhance your life. Additionally, you are preventing others you may share this information with from benefiting from it. We are all spiritual teachers; we just don't realize it or give ourselves credit for it.

Fear doesn't protect you; it limits you. It gives you a false sense of security by making you believe that if you don't put yourself out there, if you are not vulnerable, and if you don't take risks, you won't get hurt. That may be true in one sense, but you are causing yourself so much unnecessary pain by letting fear rule your life. You are eliminating the possibility of joy, wonder, and in many cases, love by living in a self-imposed locked cage. You may cry, complain, feel angry, and like a victim, when actually, you have had the key the entire time. Now is the time to use it.

END OF CHAPTER 8 QUESTIONS

1. How would you describe your life in one or two words?
2. How would you describe your health in one or two words?
3. Do you have an understanding of your life purpose or purposes?
4. What is the role of faith in your life?
5. Do you have any conditions that impact your entire body or overall quality of life?
6. Are you dealing with a life-threatening condition, or have you before?
7. Do you feel separate from the rest of the world and other people? How can you feel more connected? How can you be of more service?
8. What are the most important points you have taken from this chapter?
9. What are your spiritual and emotional symptoms associated with issues you may have in the 7th chakra?
10. Have you had a spiritual awakening?

Intuitive Sight, Wisdom, and Truth

Healing Using the 6th Chakra

Until you make the unconscious conscious, it will direct your life and you will call it fate.

—Carl Jung

Overall themes: intuitive sight,
wisdom, and truth

6TH CHAKRA

The 6th chakra is located between the eyes in the middle of the forehead and is symbolized by the color indigo. Its Sanskrit name is *Ajna* or "to perceive." This chakra is generally considered to relate to psychic and empathic experiences because it contains the "third eye" and the pineal gland. The third eye is an energy point on the forehead between your eyes. Hinduism teaches that it is the locus of occult power and wisdom in a deity, especially the god Shiva. This is one of the supreme gods who creates, protects, and transforms the universe.

Located in the middle of the brain, the pineal gland secretes melatonin, which helps to regulate circadian rhythms and, consequently, sleep. In the seventeenth century, philosopher René

Location	Physical Issues	Emotional and Spiritual Concerns
Head, brain, nose, ears, eyes Pituitary, hypothalamus Pineal gland, sinuses	Headaches and migraines Vision and hearing issues Sensitivity to mold, chemicals, scents and other toxins, touch, stimuli Brain tumor, stroke Neurological diseases or injury Seizures Learning disabilities Dementia Alzheimer's	Connection to intuition and Spirit Ability to perceive, observe, and make judgments about the world, others—too much or not enough Morality, flexibility, and need for control Ability to change and fit into society without changing so much that you lose yourself in the process Psychic ability, mood, mental illness Control vs. trusting Spirit and the universe Intelligence Spiritual awakening and emergency

Descartes claimed that this gland was the seat of the soul. Along with other parts of the brain, it has been shown to secrete DMT (N-dimethyltryptamine), a substance that can also be found in a plant called ayahuasca,[1] which is often used to trigger profoundly spiritual hallucinogenic experiences.[2]

Many people believe that the pineal gland plays a role in regulating intuition and psychic experiences, thus the 6th chakra is especially associated with these abilities.

Do you feel like you were more intuitive when you were younger? Do you remember having supernatural experiences as a child? You are not alone. Do you dream of using intuitive, healing, psychic, or creative abilities to start a business? Perhaps you just want to strengthen these abilities to help yourself or others. You don't have to be a professional intuitive or medium to have intuitive abilities or to be able to talk to the other side. We all have intuition, even medical intuition. For some of us, that skill is stronger than for others. Most of us are able to run, but some are able to run faster. Even though you may never aim to make the Olympic track team, with training and practice, you can improve your speed. It's the same with intuitive and related skills. We can all learn how to strengthen our innate abilities.

Our connection to our 6th chakra and our intuition helps us know what we think, feel, and desire. This relationship is essential if we want to be authentic. Although I don't think anyone wants to be "fake," that is exactly what we are if we change ourselves in order to be loved or approved of by others. Almost everyone who seeks my services is lost in some way and trying to get back to who they truly are. They want to return to who they were before they allowed themselves to be controlled by other people's opinions or before addiction, abuse, trauma, or illness took them off their true paths. I get it. I spent the better part of my life seeking the courage to listen to my heart and my intuition. Instead of listening to my inner voices, I looked to others for approval and love. Like most of the people I help, I have no memory of when I lost myself, but it is never too late to start over. In addressing and healing the problems of the 6th chakra, we can being to live in accordance with our authentic selves.

POSSIBLE PHYSICAL, EMOTIONAL, AND SPIRITUAL ROOT
CAUSES FOR ISSUES IN THIS CHAKRA

- Trauma
- Narcissism, personality disorders
- Anxiety, depression, addiction
- Anything that interferes with connection to intuition and spirit

- Beliefs connected to organized religion or upbringing that connects intuition and spirituality to "evil"
- Putting others' beliefs before your own, including those of cults
- Side effects of certain medications, including psychiatric meds
- Food allergies, allergies to mold, heavy metals, and pollution poisoning
- Self-doubt, low self-esteem
- Frightening experiences with the supernatural

INTUITIVE WRITING PROMPTS

- What do you want me to know about myself?
- What is blocking me from listening to my intuition?
- How is my intuition trying to get my attention?

CALL TO ACTION

If you are having any symptoms in this chakra, I believe that your intuition and Spirit are calling on you to work on them in the following ways.

PHYSICAL

Detoxify your body and environment as much as possible. If a person has a high toxicity level, even seemingly innocuous substances like vitamins or homeopathic treatments will be met by the body as invaders and cause negative side effects, thus slowing down your healing process. Certain genetic conditions and exposure to toxic substances like mold, pollution, chemical cleaners, artificial fragrances and chemicals in personal products, and pesticides can make detoxing more difficult, as can allergies to food, pets, and things in the environment.

You don't have to put yourself and your body through extensive fasts or cleanses to detox. In my experience, these can often do more harm than good, not to mention set you up for failure and self-deprivation. To begin the detoxifying process, I recommend safely getting rid of as many toxins in the environment and body as possible, to allow your immune system and adrenal glands to heal. Toxins include heavy metals, hormones, pollution, xenoestrogens (which mimic hormones), plastics, GMOs, Teflon and other non-stick coatings, and artificial fragrances. The Environmental Working Group (www.ewg.org) is an excellent source for learning about potential toxins, where they are located, and how to avoid them is. Don't forget to look at the ingredients in your makeup, skin care and hair products, deodorant, toothpaste, and sunscreen. Filtering your water for, at the very least, metals, pharmaceuticals, chlorine and chloramines (which is used even more commonly than chlorine), and fluoride is essential. Most filters are not sufficient, including most refrigerator filters, filter bottles or pitchers, and the majority of under-the-counter filters, as they do not remove chloramines and fluoride. Be selective and read the fine print when purchasing filtering systems, because even the inadequate ones can be expensive. I have a gravity-based filter on my counter with a very sophisticated ceramic filter that lasts about a year.

In addition to removing toxins from your body and the environment, you can do a modified fruit-and-vegetable fast for a couple of days, if that is workable for you; use an infrared sauna; take Epsom-salt baths (with a lot of hydration); coffee enemas (with organic coffee), if you are not allergic to coffee; use Liver Life drops from Bio Ray; and/or receive acupuncture treatments. You can also do a supervised detox with an alternative practitioner.

Don't forget your energy body. Reiki, energy treatments with a Barbara Brennan School of Healing practitioner, massage therapy, acupuncture, craniosacral therapy, lymphatic drainage, tai chi, and Kundalini yoga are only a few suggestions for ways to release damaging energy.

Emotionally, detoxing yourself from negative thoughts about yourself is crucial. Releasing anger is another important part of detoxing. It has been said that holding on to anger is like taking poison and expecting another person to die. I will say more about this in later chapters as well as in the "Condition Spotlight" later in this chapter.

EMOTIONAL

1. Do not block out the truth. Vision and hearing problems may appear because we do not want to see and hear what is actually happening.
2. Listen to and trust your intuition. Allow it to take care of you and keep you safe. Let go of micromanaging and hyper control.
3. Let go of the past and don't let trauma control you. Face your fears and do not allow yourself to be a victim. Mental illness often happens as a defense mechanism, trying to protect us from the pain of memories we think we cannot handle.
4. Do not judge yourself or others. No one is perfect.
5. Be true to yourself. Authenticity is essential.
6. Develop your intuitive and psychic abilities if you feel that you are being called to do so. There is a quiz, "Developing Your Intuitive and Psychic Skills," near the end of the chapter to help you determine the types of abilities you may have, and information on how to strengthen them.

AFFIRMATIONS AND VISUALIZATIONS FOR
THE 6TH CHAKRA

Affirmations:

- I can trust my higher self.
- I can trust my intuition.
- I can trust God and Spirit.
- I am safe and protected.
- I can see, hear, smell, touch, and taste safely.
- I can release my past and live in the present.

Visualizations:

- Visualize yourself surrounded by angels and loving spirits. You may recognize some of them or not even see their faces. Just feel the love.
- See all of your worry from the past and about the future being handed over to God, the universe, nature, or whatever feels comfortable to you.
- Imagine yourself being in the presence of whatever you might be sensitive to, such as mold, chemicals, or crowds of people, and feeling perfectly healthy and safe.

CONDITION SPOTLIGHT

AVOIDING AND PROTECTING YOURSELF FROM NEGATIVE ENERGY AND PEOPLE—EMOTIONAL CLEANSING

On social media and during work with individual clients, I often receive questions about protection from negative energy and people. There is a great fear, usually beginning in childhood, about "opening ourselves up" to negative entities and evil spirits. I also find that many people don't feel inherently safe or empowered, thinking that at any minute evil could take over their bodies or energy and that they are powerless around narcissists or bullies. Entire books have been written on this subject, discussing "energy vampires" and other such beings, but in reality, this is a very simple concept.

There are plenty of "healers" who will offer to remove evil spirits and negative attachments, sometimes requiring many appointments and at enormous cost. They tell you that you have cords attaching you to negative entities, abusive people, or even relationships from past lives, and that you are not capable or powerful enough to possibly recognize or remove them on your own. So, of course, you need to hire them to save you.

There are credible, caring people who can help release us from negative energy and beliefs and who can show us how to do that for ourselves, and I've received guidance from them in the past. However, we are not dependent on anyone else to be saved. In the same vein, while there are amazing healers who connect with Spirit and guides through a variety of methods, I know that we can heal ourselves.

I am very grateful to the practitioners I have worked with who have helped with my personal physical, emotional, and spiritual healing. We need other people, especially those who have different skill sets, insights, and abilities than we do. But healers should empower their clients and patients, not create an atmosphere of dependence. My goal is always to be part of a healing team, both personally and professionally.

We all have the ability to protect ourselves from negative energy and people. We are not just "sitting ducks" waiting to be taken over. I used to think otherwise, but I learned that with love, connection to our intuition, and by not allowing fear to take over, we are always protected and safe, even under the most frightening of circumstances.

I believe in energy, in opposites, and in the power of both good and evil. Good and love are always more powerful than evil. Negative energy uses fear to turn us away from connecting with our intuition and Spirit, because when we are fearful, we are distracted from our intuitive work and loving life purpose. One life experience in particular helped me to understand this fundamental truth and I believe it now more than ever.

The Silver Cord

At the age of seventeen, in 1983, I went away to college and soon became engaged. The marriage to Brian (not his real name) didn't last long, but he was my first serious boyfriend, the first person I felt ever actually listened or cared. At this time I was just beginning to explore my intuitive abilities; I learned that I could ask to be connected to Spirit, but I was a complete novice, learning all the time, still shocking myself with my own accuracy.

Not long after arriving at school, I had an experience I will never forget and still can't explain to this day. Around 10 P.M. one evening, Brian called, as he often did. He was six hours away from my dorm at George Washington University in Washington, DC. As we started talking, it was suddenly as if my spirit had raised from my body and traveled the hundreds of miles to where he was. I could see the dark sky and full moon outside of his window. I thought I had lost my mind, but Brian felt the same thing. It was as if I were there in person; it felt completely natural and incredibly bizarre at the same time.

Nothing like this out-of-body experience had ever happened before, and it was completely beyond my control. Eventually it felt as if I were being drawn back into my body, gently pulled along by some cord. The cord was full of light, and I couldn't tell what was on the other side. I just knew that it was bringing me back to my physical body.

Without warning, I felt intense evil. I was no stranger to evil, having grown up with it in my home, but this was more powerful than I had ever experienced. I was terrified, unable to speak or move. The closest I can come to describing it was that it was a creature clamped onto my back, literally a "monkey on my back." Its face resembled a human's, but it was anything but. I snapped out of my shock and started instinctively saying the Lord's Prayer and yelling for it to leave me alone. After what seemed like an eternity, but was probably only a few seconds, it let go and I was back in my body.

Terrifying as this experience was, it taught me a crucial lesson: it is always within our power to decide to prevent that type of energy from ever hurting us. We are always loved and protected. We are never helpless or in danger.

After this experience, my first impulse was to reject my intuitive abilities. But then I realized that my abilities were a way for me to help others, and I vowed not to allow evil and negativity to take over. I suspected that this was a way of frightening me into turning my back on my mission in life. My calling was to help others connect to their own intuition, self-love, and self-acceptance. I was not going to let evil win.

I've recalled this experience on many occasions, especially when faced with the evil behavior of members of my family or other people I have encountered. Compared to the "being" I fought off, these humans were lightweights. I can look past the false bravado and evil that makes them torment others, and see them for what they truly are: mentally ill or insecure or fearful people with absolutely no power over me.

You also have the ability to step into your own power and reject negativity and evil. You can choose to push past the people and energies that would like to suppress your goodness, and instead follow your own path with authenticity and faith.

Here are some ways to protect your energy and cleanse negative emotions and people:

- Connection to your intuition is about embracing an all-powerful loving force. Allow it to protect and guide you. You don't have to do anything except feel it's love.

- Grounding and being present are great ways to protect your energy and cleanse your emotions. Ways to ground yourself include the following:
  - Meditation
  - Being in nature
  - Mindfulness exercises and meditations that can be found on the internet (Jon Kabat-Zinn, one of the first to write about mindfulness, has some excellent ones)
  - Taking an Epsom salt bath
  - Putting your feet in a lake, pond, the ocean, or another body of water

- Make a list of all of the negative or fearful thoughts you have. If they are out of your mind and body, you can then begin to address them and release them.

- Pay attention to how you feel when you are around certain people and in certain places. Avoid ones that are draining or negative.

- See past your emotions, especially the feeling of being hurt, and look objectively at the behavior and words of those who are causing you harm. They would not mistreat others if they were healthy or if they were connected to love.

- Do not buy into a holier-than-thou or superior attitude. Some of the worst offenders I have known are people who hide behind so-called Christian values. Christ taught love and acceptance, not judgment or superiority.

- Resist the urge to try to change anyone else. You can only change your own behaviors and beliefs.

- Know that protecting yourself and your family is your right, even if it means distancing yourself or cutting off contact from other family members.

- Allow and accept your feelings, including fear. Do not push them down. Only if you bring them to the surface can you experience them, challenge them, and let them go.

- In the presence of negative or draining people, or in places that you aren't comfortable, try tools such as protective crystals, surrounding yourself with loving light, and calling in the protection of angels and Spirit.

- Always ask yourself if the emotion you are feeling belongs to you and makes sense in your world, or if you might be picking it up from someone else or somewhere else. If it doesn't belong to you, ask Spirit to return it to its owner. I find this is often the case with depression and anxiety, especially with empaths who can easily pick up the emotions of others.

- Ask yourself what the people you fear can truly do to you. What is the worst thing that can happen? Remind yourself of the times you have stood up to them and other "scary" people and have been just fine.

When you feel overcome by negativity, or find you are struggling to be true to your authentic self, take a moment to work through this grounding exercise that I learned from my friend Linda Greenleaf:

Place both feet on the floor. Standing is best but isn't required if you are not able to. Take a deep breath in, raising your arms over your head. As you do, imagine the power and love of Mother Earth coming up your legs, through the *hara* (power) line in the area of your spine, and filling your body with protective, grounding energy. As you breathe out, say to yourself, "I release all the energy, feelings, and thoughts that no longer serve me and do not belong to me." Repeat this exercise as many times as you need to feel relaxed and connected to the earth and your body.

CASE STUDY

One of my clients, "Amy," age thirty-six, contacted me for help with a number of 6th chakra issues, which were caused, in part, by the negative energy of a family member and her inability to create healthy boundaries.

6TH CHAKRA ISSUES

- Need for connection to intuition and spirit
- Desire for more authenticity (also 3rd chakra)
- Pain in the area of the head
- Sensitivity to chemicals, scents
- Anxiety
- Blurry vision

OTHER CHAKRA ISSUES

- Early trauma, grief, and loss (1st, 7th, 2nd)
- Thyroid disorder with antibodies—likely Hashimoto's (5th)
- Other autoimmune disease (1st)
- Overall dryness (7th)
- Sensitive skin (1st)
- Stress (7th)
- Very empathic, trouble with boundaries (4th)
- Alcoholism in family (1st)
- Chronic health issues that had not been adequately addressed in the past

When Amy and I spoke, she revealed that everything my guides picked up in her report was correct. Physically, her most problematic symptom was severe, debilitating migraines that had caused multiple hospitalizations and time in bed, which was taking her away from her children, whom she missed very much. She was unable to work.

We discussed her physical symptoms, which included severe migraines and extreme dryness of eyes, mouth, and skin. My guides pointed me toward an autoimmune diagnosis, specifically Sjögren's syndrome. After further testing, she was officially diagnosed with Sjögren's, and we planned out an autoimmune and anti-inflammatory diet.

Emotionally and spiritually, we focused on what was going on in her life when the symptoms started, approximately three years earlier. She had cared for her father as he suffered with lung cancer until he passed away. Her mother died a short six months later of a broken heart. Her relationship with her father had been difficult when she was younger, but fifteen years before he passed, he started attending AA, got sober, and made amends to Amy for the pain his drinking and horrible temper had caused. They had finally made their peace and became close.

Amy was mourning both her parents' deaths and the years she felt she had lost with her father. She had been pushing down her pain and grief, trying to be strong and not dwell on it, thinking it would eventually pass. Obviously, this didn't work. I taught her to talk with her intuition and the grief, allowing her painful feelings to be present without seeming overwhelming. She learned to tap into her own intuitive abilities and to speak with her parents in spirit, which brought her great comfort.

In seeking to avoid the negative energy and pain of grief, she had also been blocking out joy. The work we did together allowed her to feel everything, including the gratitude she felt for the time she had with her father while their relationship was positive, and for the love of her children and supportive husband. She reported that her migraines and other symptoms decreased dramatically and had become less severe. She felt that the spiritual healing work was just as important as the physical healing work.

DEVELOPING YOUR INTUITIVE AND PSYCHIC SKILLS

The intuitive exercises in chapter 5 are an important starting point for connecting to and strengthening your intuition, and they will also help you develop your psychic abilities. If you would like to go deeper and communicate with people who have passed, learn more about medical intuition, or strengthen your overall "spiritual knowing," you can take workshops given by mediums and healers, and there are a number of excellent books on the subject (check the appendix at the end of this book for some recommendations). But I'd also like to share some practices that have been helpful for me and my clients.

Start by taking the following quiz to learn about your intuitive and psychic skills.

TYPES OF INTUITIVE AND PSYCHIC SKILLS—WHICH DO YOU HAVE?

1. Do you remember having intuitive or psychic experiences as a child? Y or N

2. When you meet someone for the first time do you
   - A. see words in your head?
   - B. hear words in your head?
   - C. get a physical feeling?
   - D. get an emotional feeling?
   - E. not feel anything until you shake their hand or touch the person?

3. When you are in or near an old place, what happens?
   A. Nothing happens.
   B. I receive intuitive or psychic information pertaining to the building or events that happened there.
   C. I receive intuitive or psychic information pertaining to people.
   D. I have an overall positive or negative feeling.
   E. I smell things that no one else can.

4. Can you visually see spirits? Y or N

5. Can you hear the words of spirits in your head or out loud? Y or N

6. Have you seen shadows or other indications of spirit activity? Y or N

7. Do you often know something is going to happen before it does? Y or N

8. Have you felt warnings or signals about changing plans and been glad that you did? Y or N

9. Have you had vivid dreams, sometimes involving loved ones who have passed? Y or N

10. When you hold or touch objects, do you know things about where they have been, the people who have owned them, and more? Y or N

11. Can you pick up the moods of other people? Y or N

12. When you look at numbers or dates, can you see colors or hear music? Y or N

13. Do you have trouble feeling grounded and present? Y or N

14. Do you often feel anxiety or restless for no apparent reason? Y or N

15. Do you feel very connected to animals and nature? Y or N

16. Do you often feel more comfortable meditating or engaging in intuitive related activities than focused on daily life, and that you could do that forever? Y or N

17. Do you gain weight for reasons other than what you are eating, how much you exercise you do, because of hormones, or other explainable reasons? Y or N

18. When something is bothering you, is one of the first signs stomach or intestinal related issues? Y or N

19. Do you avoid watching scary movies? Y or N

20. Do you get feelings or have symptoms in your body corresponding to other people's physical symptoms? Y or N

How to Interpret the Quiz

- You may be clairvoyant, meaning that you see psychic and intuitive information, if you answered yes to 4, 6, chose A for question 2.

- You may have clairaudience, meaning that you hear information, if you answered yes to 5 and chose B for question 2.

- You may have clairsentience, meaning that you pick up intuitive information through your physical senses, if you answered yes to 10 and 18 and chose C for question 2.

- You may have claircognizance, meaning you just "know" things, if you answered yes to 7, 8, 11, 14, and 18 and chose D for questions 2 and 3.

- You may have medium abilities, meaning that you can communicate with the other side, if you answered yes to 1, 4, 6, 9, and 13 and chose C for question 3.

- You may have medical intuition, meaning that you can know information about people's health and bodies, if you answered yes to 20 and chose C for question 3.

- You may have the ability to use psychometry, meaning that you can hold or touch an object and know things about it, if you answered yes to 3 and 10.

- You may have synesthesia, which is seeing colors or hearing music when you see numbers (or a variation), if you answered yes to 12.

- You may get premonitions or have general psychic abilities if you answered yes to many of them.

TIPS FOR INCREASING YOUR PSYCHIC AND MEDIUM ABILITIES

- Practice going to historical sites and buildings, and write down what you pick up. Compare what you've written with the actual historical facts and by asking people who lived there and in the area.

- Practice with a friend. The more you practice, the more confident and accurate you become.

- Psychometry: give each other objects to see how much you can describe about their history, who owned them, etc.

- Medical intuition: have a friend give you a name and age of someone they know well, and write down what you can tell about that person.

- Have your friend think of a number or hold up a card that only he or she can see. Try to guess what the number is.

- Find a Spiritualist church in your area. Part of the service actually involves energy healing and medium readings. They often offer mediumship and other classes.

- Write down your dreams and intuitive feelings and see if any of the events come to pass.

- Talk to other people, perhaps in your family, who have had similar abilities and experiences. See if any of them compare to yours and how. You may have been having psychic and medium experiences all of your life and not realized it.

- Meditate or do a similar practice and ask for information from your guides and Spirit. Be open to what comes. Do not censor it. There are many guided meditations available at no cost online for contacting your guides and Spirit. Just put "guided meditation" into any search engine and choose what resonates.

- Spend time in nature and be open to signs and signals you receive from trees and plants as well as the earth and water. Just listen.

- Work to release stress and trauma. If you are anxious, you cannot hear anything from the other side.

- Work with others who have experience in this area who can help you feel safe and protected. If you do not feel safe, you will not be open to receive information.

- Be authentic and surround yourself with people who accept your uniqueness and your abilities.

- Review the common obstacles to connecting with intuition and psychic abilities in chapter 5.

END OF CHAPTER 9 QUESTIONS

1. What is the most frightening psychic experience you have ever had?
2. Have you ever shared this experience with anyone?
3. What fears are holding you back from connecting to your intuition and psychic abilities?
4. What can you do to counter those fears?
5. How would it change your life to trust your intuition?

6. What are the most important lessons you have taken from this chapter?
7. What are your spiritual and emotional symptoms associated with issues you may have in the 6th chakra?
8. What can you do to live a more nontoxic lifestyle?
9. Which current life situations are influencing the symptoms you are having associated with the 6th chakra?
10. Which situations in your early life are influencing the symptoms you are having associated with the 6th chakra?

Finding Your Voice

Healing Using the 5th Chakra

The most terrifying thing is to accept oneself completely.

—Carl Jung

Overall themes: expressing yourself, finding your voice, being authentic, and being vulnerable

5TH CHAKRA

This chakra is called the throat chakra and is symbolized by the color blue. The Sanskrit name is *Vishuddha,* meaning "purification." Since it is centered around the throat, the 5th chakra is commonly associated with self-expression, finding your own voice, and being heard. Sometimes problems with this chakra can manifest as overexpression—being domineering or pushing others around—but more often, people with 5th chakra issues are repressing their voices, unable to speak their minds or make themselves heard.

Issues with the 5th chakra are so common that it is rare for a client I work with to have never experienced any symptoms. It isn't a coincidence that I find more frequent and serious 5th chakra issues in women, since for so long we have been taught to push down our feelings and opinions, and

Location	Physical Issues	Emotional and Spiritual Concerns
Throat Mouth, teeth, jaw Shoulders Thyroid, parathyroid Neck and shoulders Esophagus	Hypo- and hyperthyroid, Hashimoto's and Graves' disease (autoimmune) Dental problems, gingivitis Teeth grinding Acid reflux Neck alignment, injury Rotator cuff injuries Tonsillitis Chronic sore throat Stutter Laryngitis	Self-expression—too much or not enough Will and determination Making things happen vs. waiting for things to happen Communication Authenticity, assertion Activism Trust and control Judgment and criticism Creativity

look, speak, and feel a certain way in order to make others happy. This pressure starts at a young age, with girls encouraged to be thin, not get dirty, and take care of others. I am very happy to say that this is beginning to change, as more parents, myself included, are encouraging their children to express their feelings and opinions, be creative, think differently, not follow societal norms, and to respectfully question and challenge authority. Many parents understand the serious consequences of squelching the authentic voices of their children, because they have experienced the damaging effects in their own lives.

POSSIBLE PHYSICAL, EMOTIONAL, AND SPIRITUAL ROOT CAUSES FOR ISSUES IN THIS CHAKRA

- Trauma
- Rejection, abandonment
- Lack of self-esteem
- Pushing down your feelings

- Not expressing creativity
- Not enough movement and stress relief
- Being a control freak (it's important to be able to let go and trust the universe when you need to)
- Being too strong willed and not flexible

INTUITIVE WRITING PROMPTS

- What is holding me back from feeling and expressing my feelings?
- Was there ever a time when I could be myself?
- What did my role models teach me about authenticity?
- How have unprocessed feelings influenced my emotional, spiritual, and physical health?

CALL TO ACTION

If you are having symptoms in this chakra, I believe that your intuition and Spirit are calling on you to work on the following issues if you want to attain physical, emotional, and spiritual health.

PHYSICAL

1. Thyroid: Have your levels of iodine checked. Both low and high levels of iodine can lead to thyroid dysfunction. Selenium and zinc are also important thyroid nutrients. If you suspect a thyroid issue, you can request to have your thyroid hormones tested (TSH, T4, and T3) as well as your thyroid antibodies, which can determine the presence of an autoimmune condition like Hashimotos or Graves. More information about the thyroid is available on page 116.

2. Take care of your teeth by brushing, flossing, and attending regular dental appointments. Avoid unnecessary procedures. Remove mercury fillings if you can.

3. Neck and shoulders: Stretch and move your neck and shoulders, especially if you work at a desk or look down at electronics frequently. Get massages and adjustments if you are able to. Find strengthening exercises for your shoulders if you work out, because this is a common area of injury. Shoulder pain spiritually signals "the weight of the world on your shoulders," so reduction of stress and focus on the self rather than constantly on others is very important.

4. Do not smoke or use other related products that damage your mouth, lungs, lips, or skin.

5. Pay attention to the health of your adrenal glands (for more information, see the glossary at the end of this book), since adrenal stress often impacts the thyroid.

6. If you have autoimmune disease of the thyroid, an autoimmune or anti-inflammatory diet can be very helpful.

EMOTIONAL

1. Embrace your feelings, even if you do not express them. Do not push them down. You can write them, sing them, paint them, say them to yourself—whatever method feels good to you—but do not keep them inside.

2. If you need to express yourself to someone else, do that.

3. Be authentic. Your opinion of yourself is what matters. If you are not true to yourself, your intuition will let you know. Your self-esteem will suffer, as will your physical, emotional, and spiritual bodies.

4. Be vulnerable. Allow hurt, love, and the whole gamut of emotions.

AFFIRMATIONS AND VISUALIZATIONS FOR THE 5TH CHAKRA

Affirmations:

- I am strong.
- My feelings are safe.
- I am protected.
- I am heard and seen.
- I can trust my intuition to tell me whom I can trust.
- I can safely express my creativity.
- I can leave the past behind.

Visualizations:

- Imagine expressing your feelings and opinions and being heard and respected.
- See yourself doing creative activities for fun, without worrying about the finished product.
- Visualize yourself sleeping peacefully without jaw pain or grinding your teeth.

CONDITION SPOTLIGHT

THYROID ISSUES

The thyroid gland is located in the throat and thus is associated with the 5th chakra. Many people have thyroid issues, whether it is underactive (hypothyroid), overactive (hyperthyroid), or the autoimmune conditions Hashimoto's (often a cause of hypothyroidism) and Graves' disease (often the cause of hyperthyroidism). Far too often these issues go undiagnosed because most doctors only test for thyroid stimulating hormone

(TSH) and don't test for the other thyroid hormones, such as T4, T3, or for thyroid antibodies.

I've learned from very experienced practitioners, and from my own experience, that TSH tests can come back in the normal range, even though thyroid problems are present. One issue is that a "normal" value for one person may not be normal for the next. Values on the low and high range of normal can also cause symptoms. Alternative practitioners may be much more likely to take this into account than traditional medicine practitioners.

When interpreting your numbers with TSH testing, a higher number means the opposite of what you might think, indicating lower thyroid function, while a low number means possibly overactive thyroid function. That is because more TSH is needed and thus produced when the thyroid is under-functioning. An experienced medical professional can help you understand your test results in more detail.

Thyroid dysfunction is often undiagnosed because the symptoms can be vague and mimic many other conditions. Thyroid conditions can also be caused by issues unrelated to the thyroid gland itself, like pregnancy, adrenal fatigue, some viruses, certain medications, environmental toxins like heavy metals and mold, low iodine and other nutrient levels such as ferritin (iron storage), pituitary gland dysfunction, and problems with the hypothalamus.

Autoimmune diets, careful supplementation with iodine where warranted, other supplements, stress relief to help support the adrenals, herbs, and homeopathy can all effectively help heal the thyroid.

There are a number of foods and chemicals[3] to attempt to avoid when you have thyroid disease, especially those containing goitrogens. Goitrogens are naturally occurring substances that interfere with the function of the thyroid by inhibiting uptake of iodine, which is required for thyroid health. Many of the foods in this list are healthy and people with thyroid issues usually don't have to avoid them completely. I advise trying to cut down on them to see if your body responds positively. There may be foods on the list that do not impact your thyroid at all, but negatively effect someone else's. These include:

- Soy foods: tofu, tempeh, edamame, etc.
- Certain vegetables: cabbage, broccoli, kale, cauliflower, spinach, etc.
- Fruits and starchy plants: sweet potatoes, cassava, peaches, strawberries, etc.
- Nuts and seeds: millet, pine nuts, peanuts, etc.
- Green tea in excess
- High lard intake
- Cadmium and lead
- Pesticides
- Nitrates
- Perchlorates (naturally occurring and man-made substance made of one chlorine atom and four oxygen items)
- Benzophenone (in some sunscreen and cosmetics)
- Smoking

If you are not able to heal naturally and choose to take medication, many people find that natural prescriptions, like Armour Thyroid, WP Thyroid, and Nature-Throid, work better to relieve their symptoms than artificial medications like Synthroid. But always consult with a medical professional before beginning any new prescription regimen, whether natural or otherwise.

Symbolically, issues with the thyroid reflect difficulty with expressing feelings or authenticity. I often see thyroid disease in people, especially women (who have more thyroid disease than men) who do not feel empowered in their relationships or careers. They push down their feelings and words, usually because they were not listened to, valued, or respected as children. Thyroid disease, especially autoimmune related, can run in families but genetics is not a sole determinate of health.

EXPRESSING YOUR FEELINGS TO SUPPORT YOUR THYROID

You cannot express your feelings if you don't know what they are, so the first step is allowing yourself to feel, without judgment or fear. You are probably thinking, "Easier said than done," and you are correct. One of the most difficult parts of recovery from bulimia for me was giving myself permission to feel and think, since I had become an expert at pushing everything down. I was afraid of being ridiculed by others and afraid that they would reject me or think I was weird if I allowed my true self to be seen. Too many of us have faced ridicule, rejection, anger, and even abandonment from our families and those around us starting at an early age. If the people who are supposed to love you don't accept you, how can you possibly feel safe expressing yourself alone or with strangers?

When you are in a place where you feel safe, take a moment to bring a situation or person to mind and allow yourself to feel the emotions that are tied to it—whether they come as physical sensations, thoughts, memories, or in another form. You may not feel safe allowing these emotions, especially at first, but not feeling or expressing them results in a kind of death of yourself. You begin to act, think, and feel the way you perceive how others want you to, in order to achieve love from an outside source rather than from the most important source—you. Your true feelings become buried in your body, in a place Carl Jung called our Shadow, and eventually become expressed as physical and emotional symptoms. Your self-esteem, creativity, and connection to intuition all suffer as well. You cannot live this way and be happy or healthy.

You do not have to act on or share every feeling or thought. They can just be there, in your conscious mind. Try not to judge them, just allow them. It can be very useful to work on this with the help of a therapist or trusted friend. There have been so many times in my life when I thought that what I felt or thought was weird and that I must be the only one with such a feeling, only later to find out that neither was true. Remember that people who think "differently" and in innovative ways are admired by society. These are often the same people who invent amazing things or start incredible businesses.

Once you allow your feelings and thoughts, you can decide what to do with them. You may want to just write down some of them for yourself, and you may feel compelled to share others, which might or might not be appropriate, safe, or beneficial. For example, the anger and hurt you have stored up as a result of the addictive behavior of a family member is valid, but might not even be heard or processed by that person. They likely will not change, and telling the person how you feel could make the situation even worse. Remember that your feelings do not require recognition or acceptance from another person in order to be valid. Your process of healing and stepping into your own authenticity is your journey alone and doesn't depend on the approval of others.

Regardless of how other people react, it's still important for you to process those feelings and to take action in ways that benefit you. That might be in the form of stress relief, talking to a therapist or finding a self-help group, removing yourself from the person's life or creating distance between you, along with other forms of self-care.

We often think that we can't handle the pain and fear of our feelings, but that is seldom true. You are so much stronger than you realize. The more I allowed myself emotional and spiritual growth and faced my fears, the more I realized that I had created the fear in my head. Take it one step at a time; this is a process, not an overnight accomplishment.

FAMILY SECRETS

Keeping family secrets is a common way to create and perpetuate 5th chakra issues. They do more than just withhold information or things no one talks about because they prevent everyone directly, or even indirectly, involved from being authentic and vulnerable. Whether it's the uncle who committed suicide, the mentally ill sister who was eventually committed to a mental institution, the "bachelor" cousin who never dated women, or the alcoholism that everyone pretended not to notice, family secrets are ultimately based in unnecessary shame.

These secrets not only impact the people in the generation in which they took place, but also subsequent parenting styles, relationships, and much more for many years into the future. Such was the case in my own family.

Shame and the fear of being her authentic self caused my mother to withhold a secret from almost all of the people she knew, including me, for the majority of her life. This same secret, I believe, was the spiritual root cause of her paralysis and ultimate death related to a flu vaccine reaction, because it was the only way she could escape her shame and the person who tied her to it.

I realize that vaccines can be a controversial subject, but there was no controversy or doubt that my mother's tragic condition was caused as a result of a flu shot. I bring this up because it is important to her story, and mine, because it contributed to me becoming a Medical Intuitive. I also believe that vaccines should be treated the same way as other pharmaceuticals and that we should be informed about potential side effects.

She received the shot in November 2008 and was completely paralyzed by January 2009, with milder symptoms beginning approximately a week after receiving it. She spent approximately ten years paralyzed before passing away. Her neurologists and other physicians concurred that this was a vaccine side effect after ruling out any other possible conditions and being familiar with these types of vaccine related injuries. Her doctors told us that there were several other people with similar symptoms related to flu shots, but that none of the cases were related, such as coming from the same batch. She later won her case in what is informally called vaccine court. It was created by the government after pharmaceutical companies were granted immunity from lawsuits related to vaccine injury to help with medical expenses. The cap on awards is rather low ($250K for death and emotional distress) and the majority of people who bring cases before the court are not successful. Extensive evidence of vaccine injury is required to even be granted an appearance or to have a specialized vaccine attorney accept your case.

Being our authentic selves and finding our voices aren't luxuries. They aren't things we do if we can find the time or if they don't interfere with the lives of others. They truly can be a matter of life or death.

I often tell the following story to clients who are afraid to share their truths.

The Magical Man

I don't remember how the conversation started that day in my mother's hospital room, shortly after her vaccine injury. But once she finally told me the truth, so much of my family life finally made sense. Every lie, innuendo, feeling that something just wasn't right—now I understood why. This had been a very powerful secret, and even after forty-eight years, she could barely get out the words.

"He was so magical."

"Who, Mom?"

"Your father. When I met him.

"I had just graduated from nursing school with my RN, Grace New Haven [Hospital]. It was probably May 1964, yes,

I had just graduated. I was going to start my master's program in Boston."

This was all news to me, so I was eager to learn more.

"He got serious right away. He wanted to get married and give me a ring for my birthday. I told him I wanted a stereo. I don't think he liked that."

"Probably not," I agreed. "But you got married in August of 1964, right? Why so quickly?" My mind was racing at that point, and my stomach began to tighten up.

"That summer he invited me up to Utica to meet his family."

I already knew what she was going to say.

"Did he say he was going to use a condom? Was that the first time you ever had sex?"

"Yes. I don't think he did, though."

All of my life I was told that I was born one month premature. I was born on April 15, 1965, and they got married on August 15, 1964—243 days. A normal pregnancy period is 280 days.

"You were pregnant with me when you got married? Why didn't you ever tell me? Why did you tell me all of my life that I was premature?"

"I was ashamed." My mother could barely get the words out. I will never forget the look on her face. Her voice was cracking and tears were streaming down her face. "I still am. I let Grandma and Grandpa down and felt so stupid for allowing that to happen. They were so proud of me for getting into graduate school, and I couldn't go. Even though they said I didn't have to get married and would support us, I still felt like I had no choice."

It was forty-eight years later and she could barely talk about it. My entire life was starting to make so much sense.

I finally understood why I never truly felt wanted by either one of my parents. There was always an underlying, unspoken resentment, even though my mother denied it. She was likely not even aware of it, having pushed down her feelings for so many years. I have no doubt that her shame was present every day and influenced nearly everything she did.

I left my mother's room in shock, full of so many questions that will never be answered. As a therapist I learned firsthand how much damage secrets can cause. They always end up coming out and causing far more destruction than admitting the truth in the first place would have.

My mother had shared before that she was incredibly stressed during her pregnancy. I finally understood why. The stress and shame she was forced to carry also had an effect on my emotional and physical health as an infant and on my genetics. This is called epigenetics, when our genetic expression is influenced by food, stress, and emotions. I can only imagine what feeling that intense shame every day in utero did to my genes. I know that it has made me more empathic, but since I struggled so deeply with feelings of shame when I was experiencing an eating disorder, I can't help but think there is a connection. I know that her emotions shaped my life as a child. Most of my life I felt shame and self-loathing, just like my mother. Like her, I didn't stand up for myself or take care of myself, and I often felt like a victim. I pushed anger and sadness down because I felt helpless. This is the terrible power of family secrets.

I recognized that my mother and I had rarely had an honest conversation until she became paralyzed at age sixty-five. There were the occasional glimpses of authenticity, and during those conversations she was able to admit her loneliness and unhappiness and apologize for not protecting us from my father she repeatedly told me. I could never understand why she stayed with a man who made her so unhappy and who treated her and her children so horribly. Aside from admitting to me that he had not been faithful to her, he left us alone for days at a time without explanation. He would erupt in anger at the drop of a hat and could not be depended on to show up for events or school functions and we caught him in lie after lie, not to mention the longstanding gambling addiction. My mother showed me records, that were later used in court, from the mid-1960s when he was court marshalled by the Air Force for incidents related to slot machines. I have paperwork from one of the largest casinos in the Northeast showing his losses of nearly a quarter of a million dollars. When my mother revealed the secret she'd been carrying for decades and opened up about the shame she felt, I finally understood why she couldn't leave. It wasn't that she was weak; she was broken.

Generational trauma is incredibly common. It can be transmitted by unprocessed sexual abuse or assault, mental illness, suicide, addiction, poverty, and more. Since these issues can be so difficult to talk about and are often the subjects of family secrets, you may not even realize that generational trauma has impacted your life.

The ability of people to do home DNA tests and track their genealogy has been an incredible and unexpected tool for uncovering hidden information and healing family trauma. I've had clients discover siblings they were not aware of, or that they or their parents were adopted but had never been told. When they confront loved ones with this information, it usually results in even more secrets being revealed and a deep understanding of life events and feelings they could not previously explain.

It is important to remember that we are not responsible for anyone else's actions other than our own and that what happened in the past does not have to negatively impact the future. After everything I've learned from my own experiences and my work with clients, I know that when we don't listen to our intuition and our feelings, those emotions don't just go away. Hiding the truth and suppressing our emotions simply doesn't work. The repercussions of that negative energy can be devastating for us and those around us. The only path forward is honesty and authenticity, finding the courage to use your voice and follow your intuition.

CASE STUDY

Derek, age forty-five. He contacted me regarding stress, cardiac issues, and difficult family relationships.

5TH CHAKRA ISSUES

- Difficulty allowing or expressing feelings
- Acid reflux
- Generational trauma

OTHER CHAKRA ISSUES

- High blood pressure (4th)
- Severe heart palpitations (4th)
- Fatigue and intense stress (7th)
- Difficulty concentrating (6th)
- Extra weight he was having trouble losing (3rd)
- General aches and pains (1st, 7th)
- Irritable bowel symptoms (3rd)
- Guilt and grief (7th)
- Addiction in his life and family history, primarily to alcohol (3rd, 1st)
- Relationship issues with several significant people, one of them a male (2nd)
- Being very sensitive, with empathic abilities (4th)
- Trouble connecting to and listening to intuition (6th)

Derek was on medication for the high blood pressure, which was making him even more fatigued, and he wanted to get off of it. He was using both over-the-counter and prescribed medication for acid reflux, which he had tried for years to control.

We addressed the acid reflux with various probiotics and digestive enzymes, adjusted his diet to an anti-inflammatory plan, and discussed various supplements, such as curcumin and omega-3s, which could be beneficial. We discussed strategies for gut healing and specific things he could do for stress reduction.

As we spoke, Derek revealed that he and his family were living with a family member who was having issues with health and needed care. This family member refused to allow "strangers" to come into their home to help and was very demanding, needing total control at all times. This relative was "needy" and dominated conversations, never listening to what anyone else was trying to say. Derek and his wife were confined to one part of the house, and his children stayed in their rooms, avoiding contact with the negativity. To make matters worse, this family member was an alcoholic (which my guides revealed in the report) and had been for as long as Derek could remember.

I directed Derek to the Adult Children of Alcoholics website (https://adultchildren.org/) and told him about their meetings. He had spent too long repressing his true feelings in order to survive in this difficult living situation, and he benefited from being able to talk openly about his emotions and experiences with people who truly understood. For the first time he realized that he wasn't alone. Derek hadn't considered that so many of his physical problems could be related to the intense stress and emotional impact from living with this person, silencing his own feelings, and the strain it was placing on his marriage. I taught him how to receive loving messages and guidance from within himself by connecting to his intuition. Just addressing Derek's physical issues would not have led to meaningful healing.

END OF CHAPTER 10 QUESTIONS

1. Do you feel like you can express yourself fully and be authentic? If not, with whom or under what circumstances is this most difficult?
2. Do you feel that you were seen and heard as a child? What about in important relationships and at your job? How has being seen and heard, or not, impacted your life?
3. Do you have creative outlets? How can you make more time for creativity?
4. How do you release your stress?
5. What are the most important points you have taken from this chapter?
6. What are your spiritual and emotional symptoms associated with issues you may have in the 5th chakra?
7. Which current life situations are influencing the symptoms you are having associated with the 5th chakra?
8. Which situations in your early life are influencing the symptoms you are having associated with the 5th chakra?

11

"Don't Be So Sensitive"

Healing Using the 4th Chakra

People will do anything, no matter how absurd, in order to avoid facing their own souls.

—Carl Jung

Overall themes: emotions, sensitivity, and boundaries

4TH CHAKRA

The 4th chakra is also called the heart chakra, as it is located in the area of the chest. It is symbolized by the color green. The Sanskrit name is *Anahata,* meaning "unstruck sound." This chakra is commonly associated with love and emotions, in particular with our ability to adequately express the emotions we are feeling or a tendency to take on the emotions of those around us.

The 4th chakra is one of the most common areas, along with the 3rd chakra, where emotions are often expressed as physical symptoms. It also happens to be the chakra where I most commonly pick up the presence and messages of people who have passed away in the lives of my clients when I am conducting readings.

My guides tell me that this is because I am also picking up

Location	Physical Issues	Emotional and Spiritual Concerns
Heart, circulatory system Lungs, respiratory system Breasts Upper back Shoulders Ribs	Heart disease Blood pressure—high or low Cancer of any of these areas Asthma COPD Issues related to breast health and size Pneumonia, bronchitis Congenital heart issues	Expressing emotions—too much or not enough Anger, hate, and violence Love, passion Intimacy, nurturing Grief, depression, anxiety Parenting—helicopter or neglect Giving vs. getting help Being an empath, lack of empathy Sensitivity Self vs. others—boundaries, codependency Panic attacks

the 4th chakra energy of a person who has passed—their love, worry, regrets, guilt, and their desire to connect emotionally to the person who is here and bring relief to their suffering.

POSSIBLE PHYSICAL, EMOTIONAL, AND SPIRITUAL ROOT CAUSES FOR ISSUES IN THIS CHAKRA

- Worrying about and trying to control others
- Mold, pollution, smoke, and other toxins
- Lack of ability to be vulnerable and ask for help
- Grief and loss
- Anxiety, depression, and other mental illness

INTUITIVE WRITING PROMPTS

- How do my sensitivity and empathic abilities most impact my life?

- How can I release and cope with anxiety?
- Why do I have difficulties creating healthy boundaries, and who is it most difficult to do this with?
- What am I grateful for?

CALL TO ACTION

If you are having symptoms in this chakra, I believe that your intuition and Spirit are calling on you to work on the following if you want to attain physical, emotional, and spiritual health.

PHYSICAL

1. Release stress, otherwise it is stored in the body.
2. Take care of your teeth by brushing, flossing, and attending regular dental appointments. Dental health is directly related to cardiovascular health.
3. Move your body in a way that raises your heart rate, preferably daily.
4. Do not smoke or use other related products.
5. Pay attention to the health of your adrenal glands (more about this in the glossary). Healthy adrenals help keep you from constantly being in fight-or-flight mode.
6. Eat in an anti-inflammatory manner, avoiding sugar, alcohol, processed foods, gluten, and dairy, and making most of your diet plant-based.
7. Be aware of your breathing and take deep breaths from your belly. Many people hold their breath without even realizing it.
8. Do regular self-exams of the breasts and get regularly scheduled screenings.
9. Maintain a healthy weight, since extra weight adds stress to the cardiovascular system.

EMOTIONAL

1. Regardless of whether you verbally express your feelings, allow yourself to feel them fully. Sensitivity is not a weakness or something you should be ashamed of. Take the time to process your emotions, whether that be through art, reflection, writing, or whatever method resonates with you.
2. Represent yourself authentically. Our love, passion, and empathy are all critical parts of our identities, but we are often hesitant to share them with others due to fear. Repressing your true self will only hurt you in the long term.
3. Allow people to experience negative emotions and experiences without feeling the need to save them.
4. Reflect on the advice for empaths later on in this chapter. Consider how that may apply to you and your relationships.

AFFIRMATIONS AND VISUALIZATIONS FOR THE 4TH CHAKRA

Affirmations:

- I am loved unconditionally.
- I accept myself unconditionally.
- I am beautiful.
- I can express my feelings safely.
- I can be sensitive.
- I control my energy and body and I am safe from negative energy and people.

Visualizations:

- Look in the mirror and see yourself feeling beautiful.
- Imagine loving and respecting yourself, right now.
- See yourself feeling safe in a room full of people.

CONDITION SPOTLIGHT

What Is an Empath?

Being an empath is different from having empathy. Empathy is the ability to put yourself in another person's place; it's a form of caring. Being an empath means that you often have the ability to feel another person's feelings and can be deeply impacted by them. You may have difficulty with boundaries and mistake other people's emotions for your own.

SOME OF THE COMMON TRAITS OF BEING AN EMPATH

1. Feeling the need or desire to step in and fix or save someone, especially when that person is in pain of any sort
2. Fatigue, especially in crowds or when with negative people
3. Being deeply impacted by the positive or negative moods of others
4. Taking other people's words and actions toward you personally
5. Not speaking or acting out of fear of hurting someone else's feelings
6. Feeling guilty if you impact someone "negatively"
7. Inability to establish healthy boundaries
8. Anxiety and depression from feeling overwhelmed by the world and other people as well as from trying to feel normal
9. Extreme emotional sensitivity
10. Always feeling "on" and feeling like you are walking on eggshells
11. Fear of rejection or abandonment
12. Heightened emotional response to events taking place in the world, especially negative events
13. Gut issues
14. Spending time with animals and in nature as important and healing
15. Difficulty grounding and being fully present

Advice for Empaths

1. Give yourself permission to be a separate entity. Many of us learned to be empaths as a result of having to anticipate the words and actions of others, especially when we were young. If you didn't say or do the right thing, you risked being rejected, abandoned, the wrath of someone's anger, or even abuse.

2. Learn to identify your feelings and allow them to come to the surface without judgment. It may be tempting to push down difficult or uncomfortable feelings, but that does not make them go away. Rejecting your feelings will only make them stronger and gives them more power over you.

3. Ask yourself if your painful or uncomfortable feelings belong to you, if they make sense in your world and in your circumstances, or if you might be picking them up from someone else or from the collective mood of a group. If your feelings are personal and are related to things within your control, start taking concrete steps to address them, like talking to a therapist or changing your life circumstances, such as where you live, your relationships, or your job. If the feelings are a result of something you cannot control, such as world events or the behavior and circumstances of another person, recognize that you cannot control them, and take steps to release them, such as physical exercise, mindfulness meditations, therapy, or creative pursuits. If they are being picked up from outside of yourself, actively release them into the universe or to God. You can write down your feelings and put them into a box, burn the paper, or visualize yourself sending them off into space.

4. Do not hesitate to ask for help with your feelings from a qualified therapist, especially if being empathic was learned as a result of trauma or a dysfunctional childhood.

5. Learn to express your feelings and opinions and establish healthy boundaries. Refer back to the previous chapter for advice on how to start owning and expressing your feelings. Connection to intuition can help with this immensely, as I discussed in chapter 5.
6. Learn to recognize signals and symptoms from your body. I will address this more in the following chapter, but stomachaches, heart palpitations, headaches, digestive and intestinal issues, and other symptoms often happen as a result of our own emotions and picking up the feelings of others. These symptoms may happen long before we realize what we are even feeling.
7. Remember that you control your own energy, so you do not have to fear negative energy or picking up negativity from others. You also don't have to rely on anyone else to "remove" negative energy. If you notice yourself feeling sad, depressed, or angry in the presence of another person or in a specific environment, first be aware and embrace your feelings. If these feelings do not belong to you, simply give them back to the person or to the universe. Set up boundaries of love and light around yourself and decide how you want to feel.

Even extremely sensitive people can do these things. Much of the time emotional sensitivity is difficult because you may have trouble tolerating other people being in pain. This is often about you, not the other person. The other person's pain likely brings up recollections of your own suffering or trauma. I was so sensitive as a child that I sobbed for five hours after watching a cartoon about a pair of Canada geese that had mated for life. A hunter killed one of them, and I couldn't stop thinking about the intense grief the survivor must have felt. Crying over a cartoon wasn't rational and I knew it, but I couldn't stop.

As a very sensitive person, you may feel the need to "fix" or soothe, which is absolutely normal and caring. However, being there for someone if they *ask* for your help is different from imposing your thoughts, beliefs, and feelings on someone else. We learn from pain, and if you try to prevent someone from feeling it, they may be missing out on incredibly significant learning and growth experiences.

It is common for me to see 4th chakra symptoms, especially cardiovascular disease and breast cancer, in people who are extremely sensitive and who easily pick up the feelings and energy of others. Sensitivity and especially empathic traits are usually developed at a very young age, as survival responses to a dysfunctional environment where you could never predict what would happen next. I also commonly see 4th chakra symptoms in people who spend much of their time "fixing," "mothering," or trying to control other people, including helicopter parenting.

CASE STUDY

Caroline, age thirty-seven, who was looking for help with respiratory issues and managing trauma and stress.

4TH CHAKRA ISSUES

- Trauma, grief, and loss
- Sensitive and empathic
- Heaviness in the chest, difficulty taking deep breaths
- Frequent respiratory infections

OTHER CHAKRA ISSUES

- Need for connection to intuition and Spirit (6th, 7th)
- Desire for more authenticity, female power connection (2nd, 3rd)
- Sensitive skin (1st)

- Sensitivity to chemicals, scents, mold (6th)
- Stress, anxiety (6th, 7th)
- Substance abuse in family (3rd)
- Chronic health issues that had not been adequately addressed in the past

When Caroline and I spoke, she shared that she had contacted me because of recurrent respiratory infections and difficulty taking deep breaths.

We discussed possible physical reasons for the respiratory issues, such as mold exposure and allergens. She confirmed that this had been an issue in her home. We talked about homeopathic remedies to help her detox from mold, and I offered to refer her to a naturopath. We also worked on strategies to naturally strengthen her immune system, dietary changes, and ways to address better nutrient absorption.

We discussed stress reduction and anxiety reduction strategies, since her chest tightened up when she felt out of control. She had a history of panic attacks, with rapid heartbeat as well. These occurred sporadically in her late twenties and early thirties but increased with the onset of her other symptoms.

Emotionally and spiritually, we focused on what was going on in her life when the symptoms started five years ago. She caught her husband having an affair after suspecting it for several months. She found romantic texts on her husband's phone from her neighbor, who was one of her closest friends. The affair had been going on for ten months. She said that when she read the texts, her chest tightened up and she felt like she couldn't breathe. She experienced one of the most intense panic attacks of her life.

Her husband did not attempt to deny the affair, and they decided to work to save the marriage, but Caroline was having doubts about whether she could ever trust him again, let alone her own intuition.

She had been pushing down her pain, fear, and grief, trying to be strong and not dwell on it, thinking it would eventually pass, but the feelings only grew. Her emotions were making themselves felt as physical symptoms relating to her 4th chakra, literally making it hard to breathe and crushing her with anxiety. She and her husband were attending counseling, but I pointed out that she needed a place to focus on herself and her own feelings, separate from the marriage. We worked on building her connection to intuition, self-love, and taking more time for herself, rather than always thinking about others. We explored her honest feelings about the problems in her marriage, and eventually she decided that a separation would be best. Fortunately, her husband was willing to move out of the house and amicably co-parent their two children.

The more empowered she felt, the less frequently her panic attacks occurred and breathing became easier.

We worked on helping her to feel empowered and to express her feelings and feminine energy through creativity, yoga, and dance. We also talked about the kind of work she wanted to be doing and the pursuit of her passions in life, which meant changing careers. She decided she would go back to school and finish her master's degree in art therapy.

END OF CHAPTER 11 QUESTIONS

1. If you have experienced trauma, how do you think that has impacted your ability to feel and express emotions?
2. What symptoms alert you to the need to allow and express your emotions, or that you are picking up the emotions of others?
3. How do you release stress?
4. What were the most significant parts of this chapter for you?

5. What are your spiritual and emotional symptoms associated with issues you may have in the 4th chakra?
6. Which current life situations are influencing the symptoms you are having associated with the 4th chakra?
7. Which situations in your early life are influencing the symptoms you are having associated with the 4th chakra?

12

Self-Esteem, Body Image, and the Gut-Brain

Healing Using the 3rd Chakra

The greatest tragedy of the family is the unlived lives of the parents.

—Carl Jung

Overall themes: self-esteem, caring for oneself, and instinct and intuition

3RD CHAKRA

Located between the navel and the base of the breastbone, the 3rd chakra is also called the solar plexus and is symbolized by the color yellow. It's Sanskrit name is *Manipura,* meaning "city of jewels." It is connected to the gut, including "gut feelings" and intuition, as well as to themes of self-esteem and self-care.

The 1st, 2nd, and 3rd chakras are where I commonly see the most symptoms. I believe that this is because these chakras are most impacted by childhood experiences and trauma. I rarely encounter someone who has had a "happy" childhood with caring parents. Our upbringings set the stage for not only our root (1st) chakra health related to basic needs, safety, and

Location	Physical Issues	Emotional and Spiritual Concerns
Upper intestines Stomach Liver Adrenals Gallbladder Kidneys Spleen Pancreas	Gut inflammation, IBS, leaky gut Bacterial imbalance Food intolerances Ulcers Liver disease Addiction Adrenal fatigue, cortisol Weight concerns Diabetes Bowel issues, Crohn's, constipation	Addiction Eating disorders Self-esteem—not enough or narcissism Responsibility to yourself vs. others Self-care Perfectionism, ability to take criticism Pride—too much, not enough Body image, body dysmorphia

security, but also the 2nd chakra, centered around relationships, life purpose, and creativity, and the 3rd chakra, related to self-esteem, authenticity, addiction, and body image. I am happy to report that the vast majority of clients I work with are actively raising their children differently than they were raised and are working on breaking the cycle of dysfunction, addiction, and trauma.

Both the immune system and nervous system are directly connected to the gut, so it shouldn't come as a surprise that 3rd chakra symptoms are some of the most common complaints I pick up. The gut is also called the "second brain" because so many emotions are picked up and processed here and because the majority of neurotransmitters (the chemicals that control and mitigate emotions) are made here by gut bacteria. These neurotransmitters include serotonin, norepinephrine, GABA, and dopamine. In addition, your gut contains approximately five hundred million neurons, which are connected to your brain through nerves in the nervous system.

One of the largest nerves is the vagus nerve, which modulates the stress response. Studies have shown that stress reduces the strength of the signals through the vagus nerve and, as a result, causes gastrointestinal problems, including irritable bowel syndrome and Crohn's disease.

A huge proportion of the immune system is in your digestive tract, including cells in the lining that produce important antibodies. Researchers are still in the process of understanding how and why these antibodies are created and of determining the varieties of these important compounds, along with exactly how the proper bacterial balance in our gut influences our overall health. Sadly, the importance of gut health is a relatively new topic by mainstream practitioners. However, naturopaths, Chinese medicine including acupuncture, Ayurveda, and other so-called alternative health providers have been stressing the importance of gut health and food as medicine for centuries. All of these critical health factors—the gut, immune system, and nervous system—are tied to the 3rd chakra.

POSSIBLE PHYSICAL, EMOTIONAL, AND SPIRITUAL ROOT CAUSES FOR ISSUES IN THIS CHAKRA

- Unresolved emotions, including anger and fear
- Addiction
- Toxins (Guillain-Barré syndrome, the paralyzing autoimmune disease that took my mother's life, often originates in the gut from reaction to toxins, including food poisoning.)
- Being empathic, lack of proper boundary setting
- Improper nutrition or difficulty absorbing nutrients
- Body image issues
- Parasitic infection
- Bacterial imbalance (too much unhealthy bacteria)
- Virus, including chronic viruses
- Bacterial infection
- Organ disease or injury, such as gallbladder, stomach, or liver

INTUITIVE WRITING PROMPTS

- How can I allow more self-love? What is blocking it?
- What emotions/situations cause me to eat when I am not hungry or to lose my appetite?
- Is the way I see my body the same or different than the way others see it? Do I have body dysmorphia?

CALL TO ACTION

If you are having symptoms in this chakra, I believe that your intuition and Spirit are calling on you to work on the following if you want to attain physical, emotional, and spiritual health.

PHYSICAL

1. Stress can be stored in the body, so it's important to find ways to release it and promote peace.
2. Address addiction related behaviors and thoughts. If you are not doing this already, twelve-step programs and support groups related to addiction and growing up in a family with addiction issues, such as Alcoholics Anonymous, Narcotics Anonymous, Al-Anon, and ACOA (Adult Children of Alcoholics) are great places to start.
3. Address gut health using appropriate probiotics for your conditions to balance bacteria, take in adequate fiber (at least twenty-five to thirty grams from food per day), and drink water to adequately hydrate for healthy bowel function.
4. Avoid overusing or misusing Tylenol and other medications that can be dangerous to the liver.
5. Maintain a healthy weight and eat intuitively. Diets don't work long term, and repetitive dieting can have detrimental effects on metabolism and hunger/thirst messages. More about this later in the Condition Spotlight of this chapter.

EMOTIONAL

1. Listen to and honor your own instincts. Our "gut feelings" are not random whims, but important messages from intuition. Be as authentic as possible.
2. Work on healing trauma and releasing outdated, negative messages you have heard from others and have told yourself.
3. Pay attention to gut-related symptoms. Many people, especially empaths, pick up emotions and feel stress in the gut area. Your physical symptoms may have emotional and spiritual root causes.

AFFIRMATIONS AND VISUALIZATIONS FOR THE 3RD CHAKRA

Affirmations:

- I am enough.
- I am perfect exactly the way I am.
- I am beautiful and loved.
- My body is my friend.
- I love my body.
- The food that I eat is healthy and nourishing.
- I can trust my intuition.

Visualizations:

- Imagine eating whatever you would like without guilt or shame.
- Visualize feeling comfortable in your own skin doing something you have been self-conscious about doing.
- See yourself being free of addictive thoughts and behaviors.

CONDITION SPOTLIGHT

WEIGHT, BODY IMAGE, AND CHRONIC DIETING

Weight. *Ugh.*

What we weigh isn't only about calories in, calories out. Our weight is also influenced by our personal feelings and behaviors regarding self-protection, taking in other people's feelings, grounding, storing of emotions, self-esteem, blood sugar, heredity, damage we may have done to our metabolism, and countless other factors. These correspond to the physical and emotional components controlled by the 3rd chakra.

I had literally spent every waking minute from age twelve until my early twenties, obsessing about every pound, every calorie, every morsel of food, drop of water, how much I pooped, and more. You name it, if it had to do with my weight, it was on my mind. That changed after I lost twenty pounds shortly after beginning Prozac and was able to keep it off without dieting or restricting food. This experience completely changed what I had previously thought about weight.

The obsessive thoughts and behaviors started long before I developed a full-blown eating disorder. The day my father told me that I was too fat to eat ice cream and I decided to go on a diet, my life changed permanently. I vividly remember seeing myself and my body differently. A switch flipped and there was suddenly something wrong with me, a lie I told myself for decades after.

I have been helping people with the complex issues of body dysmorphia (seeing yourself differently than how you actually look), eating disorders, and weight issues for over thirty years. Some common reasons why people may lose touch with their body related to weight and food include: feeling in control for the first time when dieting and losing weight; having weight loss or overeating spiral out of control because of sports, relationships, trauma, stress, or peer pressure; or having parents (often mothers) who modeled unhealthy behavior regarding weight and food. No matter the specific details, the root causes are exactly the same: low self-esteem, shame, lack of ability to be one's authentic self, and missing connections with Spirit and intuition.

I was very cognizant of this while raising our daughters but still made mistakes. I hadn't been bulimic for many years and was at a healthy weight by the time our first daughter was born, but I thought (and talked) about my weight and what I ate far too frequently. Even though I vowed that I would not "pass on" my eating disorder, and that I wanted my children to feel confident and to love their bodies, I still managed to create an atmosphere in which one of my daughters picked up a preoccupation with healthy eating, weight, and developed an eating disorder of her own.

Through her recovery, she introduced me to a book called *Intuitive Eating* by Elyse Resch and Evelyn Tribole, which I often recommend to clients. Many of the ideas are essentially the same concepts I initially worked through with my therapist as I was recovering from bulimia. Principles such as letting your body tell you what it wants and needs, letting your body get to its natural weight, eating mindfully, moving for fun, etc. The intuitive eating movement also reveals how people work against themselves by dieting and obsessing about what they weigh. The less we eat, the lower our metabolism becomes because our bodies enter starvation mode.

Our bodies inevitably change with time as our hormones shift. My body has changed considerably since I turned fifty and went into menopause. I gained weight around my middle and back, where I never had it before, and I'll admit that I wasn't happy about it. I did what always worked for me before, altering my diet and exercising more, but that didn't work. The more I exercised, the higher the number on the scale became, but the weight gain wasn't fat, it was muscle. I had to come to terms with my new, larger, stronger body, and I have learned to embrace it. My younger daughter says that "it is okay to take up space." She is very wise.

If I were to tell you that I have this weight and body-image thing entirely figured out, I'd be lying, but I have made light-years of progress. I'm happy to say that I have healed considerably and have had a great deal of success helping others.

Here are some of the most important things I've learned about weight loss and healthy weight maintenance:

- If you would like to lose weight, realize that diets don't work long term. The more you diet, the lower your metabolism will become and the fewer calories your body will need to maintain the same weight. You also lose muscle unless you are doing weight-bearing and weight-building exercises, which means that your body is burning fewer calories. As we get older, the amount of muscle in our body naturally decreases unless we actively build it, so our metabolism goes down with it. Accept these natural changes and work with your body instead of against it. Rather than going on a "diet," think about making lasting lifestyle changes, like listening to your body's signals about hunger, thirst, being full, and wanting to move. Think back to when you were a child, before you started eating for emotional reasons and exercised just to lose weight, before food brought connotations of guilt and shame.

- Work on strengthening and supporting your adrenal glands with stress relief, adequate rest, and sleep (see additional information about this in part 2 for further suggestions). When we're stressed, our adrenal glands produce excess cortisol, which signals our bodies to store fat, unrelated to the number of calories consumed.

- The less we eat, the less we feel our hunger, which complicates the problem. I've actively had to remind myself to eat more because I tend not to take in enough calories, even though I'm not dieting. It's a bit of a tricky concept because

I don't want to eat if I'm not hungry, but I need enough fuel for the amount of physical activity I engage in. Learn to pay attention to your own hunger cues and honor what your body is telling you without judgment.

- Exercise helps to stimulate both your appetite and your metabolism. It also reduces anxiety, which many women have connected to weight and eating, so I can't recommend it highly enough. Find something you truly love. For me that is pole dancing. I don't even think about "exercising" or weight when I am pole dancing. I look forward to every class, the challenge it provides, and the group of supportive, amazing people I have the pleasure of spending time with. Find ways to move that you love!

- Get off the scale. If you need a measure of health, have your body composition measured professionally. Fat, muscle, and water percentages are much more accurate representations of the state of your body than numbers on a scale.

- Ask your body and intuition about the symbolic nature of extra weight on your body. When I am not listening to my intuition, not practicing enough self-care, or allowing anxiety over the past or the future to take over my thoughts, it isn't uncommon for me to gain weight. Symbolically, weight is a way of grounding us and getting our attention. Rather than panicking or feeling bad, talk to your body and consider what the extra weight is communicating. You can use the same writing technique for this as the one I taught you in chapter 5. I often will ask if the weight is a signal from my intuition, what that signal is, and what feelings I might be pushing down.

- Addressing trauma and fear is essential. I know that my relationship with my body changed after I was bullied, and this directly contributed to the development of the eating disorder. Work with a qualified therapist, preferably one who helps you to connect with intuition, so that you can move forward without the negative messages, fear, and shame that abuse, assault, bullying, or other trauma often creates.

- Try not to think of foods as "good" or "bad," as this can trigger guilt and shame. Food can directly impact mood, health, and the immune system, so, yes, it is important to eat as healthily as possible to optimize nutrients, but it's also okay and necessary to eat foods that are fun and taste good. When you are recovering from dieting (yes, that is a thing) or an eating disorder, restricting or limiting foods can be triggering. Listen to what your body truly wants, chew it slowly so that you can taste it, and process the experience and listen to how it feels in your body once you have eaten it. If it isn't delicious, don't bother eating it. If it creates any negative effects, it is likely not best for *your* body and you might want to avoid it.

EATING DISORDERS

These are characteristics of disordered eating as defined by the DSM-5 (*Diagnostic and Statistical Manual of Mental Disorders,* fifth edition), which is the American Psychiatric Association's "bible" for diagnosis, often for purposes of insurance and consistent labeling. Most disordered eating doesn't fit neatly into one box, and often a person starts out with one set of symptoms and graduates to more severe symptoms like bulimia or anorexia. You may recognize yourself in more than one of these categories. I've modified the language to make it more user-friendly.

Anorexia Nervosa

A. Restriction of calories leading to a significantly low body weight
B. Intense fear of gaining weight or becoming fat, or persistent behavior that interferes with weight gain, even though at a significantly low weight

C. Unrealistic perceptions of body weight, like thinking you are "fat" when you are at a healthy weight or weight that is too low for your height

Bulimia Nervosa

A. Recurrent episodes of binge eating, which is defined as consuming an excessive amount of food in a short period of time, far more than what natural hunger would normally allow; also feeling a lack of control while eating
B. Using self-induced vomiting, laxatives, diuretics, or other medications, fasting, or excessive exercise to try to lose or maintain weight
C. Binge eating and negative behaviors to prevent weight gain, both occurring, on average, at least once a week for three months
D. Self-evaluation unduly influenced by body shape and weight

Binge Eating Disorder

This disorder has the same characteristics as for bulimia but without the purging behavior.

Orthorexia

Orthorexia isn't officially recognized by the American Psychiatric Association as an eating disorder, but in my opinion it should be. It is a term coined by Steven Bratman, MD, to describe his own experience with food and eating. It literally means "fixation on righteous eating." It often starts as an attempt to be healthier and even lose weight, but it eventually becomes an obsession with calorie and nutrient counting, food restriction, exercise, perfection, and extreme judgment of the self and others who are not as obsessed or concerned with health and weight. Self-esteem becomes based on health and the ability to maintain this rigid lifestyle.

IDENTIFYING DISORDERED EATING—SIGNS AND SYMPTOMS

Eating disorders can manifest in many different ways, but these are some common signs and behaviors that might be cause for concern:

- Feeling unsettled or anxious after eating, needing to exercise or eliminate what you just ate
- Keeping track of calories, nutrient grams, and how many calories you burn, either on paper or in your head
- Constant thoughts about food, fat, and weight; frequently weighing yourself
- Self-esteem and mood based on weight, size, adherence to a diet, how you look compared to others
- Feeling anxiety, guilt, or shame if you do not exercise, especially after eating
- Regularly eating for reasons other than hunger, including sadness, anxiety, or shame; not connecting emotions with eating or allowing yourself to feel; eating as a coping mechanism to avoid feeling anything at all
- Frequent comparisons of your body and weight to others
- Believing that you cannot or should not do something because of size or weight
- Feeling self-conscious eating around others

ADDRESSING ISSUES ABOUT FOOD AND YOUR BODY

It's often necessary to seek professional help for eating-disordered thoughts and behaviors. I could not have gotten better on my own and wish I had sought help earlier. I strongly recommend therapy and treatment that has a spiritual, intuitive component. Many models are strictly behavior-based, and from my experience, this isn't very effective.

These programs, especially inpatient ones, put an emphasis on control, usually relinquishing it to others rather than listening to oneself. People with eating disorders often struggle with control as part of the disease. These people frequently come from controlling, dysfunctional families, so I don't think it is therapeutic in most cases to take away control and have people earn "privileges," such as phone calls or privacy, if they gain weight and otherwise conform. Although, I do agree that there may be cases in which this type of treatment is temporarily warranted, such as when someone's life is in danger if they do not gain weight.

I fully believe that I would not have recovered if I had not learned to talk with and trust my intuition, learned to love and accept myself, and learned how to separate from my dysfunctional family. Jungian counseling made this possible because it stresses these concepts, along with helping you change and modify your behaviors and thought patterns. It uses art therapy and symbolism to help extract thoughts and feelings that people with eating disorders learn to push down, and also to help heal trauma, which is a common root cause of disordered eating.

Medication such as antidepressants may be helpful for changing brain chemistry issues that contribute to eating disorders. I do not believe that medications should be used long term or as the sole form of treatment if they can be avoided, however, there is absolutely no shame in using them if you need to. Before taking them, I recommend that you educate yourself about side effects, as many antidepressants cause weight gain, which can provoke anxiety and be counterproductive to treatment. I can't tell you the number of times I have had clients prescribed antidepressants with this side effect, only to have them progress further into their disorder.

Whether you have a full-blown eating disorder or if, like most women and an increasing number of men, you are not comfortable with your body, aren't sure how to listen to your body's signals about eating and movement, and/or are overwhelmed and confused about the amount and accuracy of information available regarding food, exercise, and weight, it is important to work on seeing yourself as more than a number on a scale or as an object that must be and look perfect. Get to know your authentic, true self, prioritizing what you feel and think rather than basing your life on what other people think. Let go of an artificial sense of control, address anxiety, and come to terms with being sensitive, a trait I have found that many eating-disordered people share. Sensitivity is lovely as long as we create boundaries between ourselves and others.

Long-standing habits, often learned early in life, can be hard to break. These are some strategies that can help:

- Body dysmorphia, or distorted body image, is an incredibly common problem, whether you are perceiving yourself to be larger or smaller than you actually are. A great way to check your beliefs against reality is to try this art therapy exercise: Get a large roll of brown or white paper from a craft or art supply store. Spread it out on the floor or tack it on a wall at a length greater than your height and wider than your body. If the paper is not wide enough, tape two pieces together. Ask a trusted friend, therapist, or family member to trace around your body with a marker or pencil, hugging the curves of your body to get as accurate a representation as possible. Compare your body tracing to the image of your body you have in your head. When I did this exercise myself, I remember being amazed at how much smaller I was than what I was perceiving in the mirror.

- Think about how the people you were raised by, or who otherwise influenced you at an early age, thought and spoke about food, weight, and self-esteem. What did you learn, and how did it influence your thoughts and behaviors?

- Consider how you think and feel about food and your own body. Identify messages you send yourself and write them down, both positive and negative. What messages are you giving to your own children? Ask them, if you aren't sure.

- Keep a diary for a few days or a week about what you eat (or when you don't want to eat), when you exercise or don't, and most importantly, your feelings during this time. See if you can identify any patterns and recurring themes. Use these as topics to work on during therapy or your own intuitive work.

- Put away the scale and make a commitment to try to compare yourself to others less. Also make a commitment to pass by your image in a mirror or window without analysis and criticism. You don't have to do this for a lifetime: try a week at first and notice how you feel.

- Purchase some clothes that fit you well and that are flattering, ideally ones that don't hide your shape behind bagginess or folds. How many of us have put off buying new clothes until we "lose weight," wearing clothes instead that aren't flattering and make us feel unattractive. You don't have to earn the right to look and feel confident by losing weight. If you shop at a discount store or consignment shop, this doesn't have to cost much money.

- Make a list of what you would do "if you lost weight." It might be to go swimming in public, start a business, initiate sex or have it with the lights on, start a new relationship, ask for a promotion, or make presentations in front of others at your job. Stop waiting to live. Take steps to start following your dreams today, even if they are baby steps.

This is just a very short overview of eating disorders, body image, and paths to healing, but hopefully it will help you begin to find balance and a new relationship with yourself and your body.

CASE STUDY

Since I have written extensively about eating disorders, I want to present a case study about a woman I worked with, Claire, age forty-seven, who was struggling with other addictions (connected to the 3rd chakra), namely alcohol, cigarettes, and shopping.

3RD CHAKRA ISSUES

- Personal addiction issues—alcohol, cigarettes, and shopping
- Shame, body dysmorphia
- Poor nutrition and malabsorption of nutrients
- Gut imbalance, gut symptoms

OTHER CHAKRA ISSUES

- Inadequate stress relief (7th)
- High-stress job, difficult marriage (2nd)
- Intolerance to chemicals, fragrances (6th)
- Difficulty expressing emotions (4th)
- Acid reflux (5th)
- Anxiety, grief (4th, 6th)
- Dysfunctional family history with substance abuse (1st)

- Asthma as a child (4th)
- Intense sensitivity and empathic abilities (4th)
- Hormonal symptoms—difficulty sleeping, general fatigue, weight changes (2nd, 3rd, 7th)

My guides had given me information about Claire's grandmother who had passed away five years earlier. Claire was closer to her grandmother than any other family member and was still grieving her death but wasn't fully aware of how much the grieving was impacting her, until we discussed it.

Claire confided that the main reason she contacted me was for help with alcohol addiction, depression, and anxiety. She was also unhappy with recent weight gain and an inability to lose it. We talked about the impact of her loss and the signals that her body and Spirit were giving her about needing more stress relief, allowing her feelings to surface and be released, and connection to intuition so that she could love and accept her true self. Her grandmother was the only person she felt that she could relax with and be accepted by.

We discussed her marriage, which she entered into in her early twenties and hadn't been happy with for the past ten years. She knew she had to get out but was putting it off "until she felt better emotionally and physically." I pointed out that she was likely using alcohol as a way to squelch her feelings of shame, guilt, emotional abandonment by her husband, as well as the anger she felt at herself for putting up with her husband's emotional abuse and lack of affection. Believing that she could wait to leave the relationship was not realistic because she wouldn't be able to heal emotionally or physically unless she was free from the negativity of her marriage.

We discussed taking first steps toward divorce, like following through with the attorney she consulted last year, looking for another place to live, and telling her children. We designed a nutritional plan to help her body create additional neurotransmitters and increase energy, and I suggested she investigate a number of supplements and minerals, including those that support liver health, reduce her cravings for alcohol, and curb acid reflux.

I encouraged her to join a twelve-step program for addiction as well as to start attending Adult Children of Alcoholics (ACOA) meetings.

I can happily report that Claire is now divorced and living in a place she loves. After a few stops and starts, she has maintained her sobriety for over a year and is now sponsoring others at ACOA. Her acid reflux is gone, and her gut symptoms have been greatly reduced, only flaring if she is anxious. She is able to talk with her intuition and recognize which feelings are hers and which she may be picking up from other people.

END OF CHAPTER 12 QUESTIONS

1. Did you identify with the section on disordered eating? What traits did you pick up about yourself?
2. Do you have gut symptoms associated with your emotions or the emotions of others? Which ones? Try putting away the scale for a month and pay attention to how you feel.
3. Are you a perpetual weigher or dieter? If so, what have been the effects on your mind and body?
4. What foods or ingredients does your body seem to react negatively to? How did you discover this?
5. Do you have addictive behaviors or tendencies? What are they, and how have they impacted you?
6. Where did your beliefs about food and weight come from? In what ways do images and words in the media impact how you feel about how you look?
7. What are your spiritual and emotional symptoms associated with issues you may have in the 3rd chakra?

8. Which current life situations are influencing the symptoms you are having associated with the 3rd chakra?
9. Which situations in your early life are influencing the symptoms you are having associated with the 3rd chakra?

13

Sex, Power, and Life Purpose

Healing Using the 2nd Chakra

I am not what happened to me, I am what I choose to become.

—Carl Jung

Overall themes: relationships versus career, balance of feminine/masculine energy, sexuality, creativity

2ND CHAKRA

The 2nd chakra is also called the sacral chakra and is symbolized by the color orange. It's located below the navel in the pelvic region and is commonly associated with sexual energy, inspiration, and creativity, and can often reflect experiences of trauma or shame. In Sanskrit, it is called *Svadhisthana,* meaning "sweetness."

As I have said, emotional and spiritual issues are commonly expressed as physical symptoms, and I find that this is frequently the case in this area of the body. Symptoms of the 2nd chakra can be embarrassing, shameful, emotionally charged, and difficult to talk about and diagnose because they relate to the sexual organs and organs related to expelling waste. It is

Location	Physical Issues	Emotional and Spiritual Concerns
Sex organs	Fertility	Feminine/masculine
Bladder	PMS	energy balance
Prostate	Endometriosis, fibroids	Abuse trauma
Hips, hip flexors	Polycystic ovary	Creativity
Lower back	syndrome	Career and work vs.
Large intestine	Interstitial cystitis,	personal time
	urinary problems	Intimacy
	Hormone imbalance	Sexual expression and
	Menopausal symptoms	pleasure, orgasm
	Sexual dysfunction	Body image and body
	Back pain	dysmorphia
		Anxiety about future

very helpful for me to detect and label issues in general in my report and painting before speaking with clients, especially 2nd chakra issues, because it isn't uncommon for clients to be talking about these issues for the very first time or to not even be fully aware of them. Bringing them up first "breaks the ice" and makes the experience of discussing and processing them easier. I have also found my experience as a licensed counselor to be quite valuable in these circumstances.

POSSIBLE PHYSICAL, EMOTIONAL, AND SPIRITUAL ROOT CAUSES FOR ISSUES IN THIS CHAKRA

- Lack of identification and expression of female/male power; imbalance of masculine/feminine energy in life and self
- Shame regarding sexuality, sexual identity
- Lack of creative expression
- Dissatisfaction with career, life-path process
- Disappointment/unhappiness with romantic relationships and friendships
- Body image issues
- Inability to be intimate, vulnerable

INTUITIVE WRITING PROMPTS

- What coping strategies have I used to help protect myself and heal from trauma?
- How do I feel about sex, and what events/beliefs shape how I feel?
- If I could wave a magic wand, what would I like to do with my life?

CALL TO ACTION

If you are having symptoms in this chakra, I believe that your intuition and Spirit are calling on you to work on the following if you want to attain physical, emotional, and spiritual health.

PHYSICAL

1. Release stress, otherwise it is stored in the body.
2. Attend to the health of your reproductive system with regular exams, etc.
3. Stretch and strengthen your back, core, and hips.
4. Allow and embrace physical sexual pleasure.
5. Pay attention to hip and hip flexors, working on stretching and mobility.

EMOTIONAL

1. Explore your feelings and beliefs about what it means to be sexy. Do you associate it with positive feelings or shame, guilt, and pornography?
2. Be authentic. Don't repress your own creativity, and express yourself without inhibition. Be honest about your desires and curiosities sexually and approach them without shame.

3. Allow yourself to be intimate and explore reasons why you may push people away.

4. Work on healing trauma and releasing outdated, negative messages you have heard from others and have told yourself.

AFFIRMATIONS AND VISUALIZATIONS FOR THE 2ND CHAKRA

Affirmations:

- I can have a healthy relationship.
- I can express myself safely through my creativity.
- I can let go of and heal from trauma.
- I am safe and protected.
- I can trust my intuition.
- I can let go of guilt and shame.
- No one can ever hurt me again.

Visualizations:

- See yourself letting go of traumatic memories. Give them to God, the angels, the ocean, or whatever feels comfortable.
- Imagine being in a relationship where you feel loved, appreciated, and respected.
- Visualize being in a job you love or starting your own company.

Two important issues I encounter frequently are sexual assault or abuse and the PTSD that often follows traumatic events like these. PTSD can apply to every chakra, depending on the nature of the trauma it has resulted from, and because it impacts every part of our lives: physically, emotionally, and spiritually. Sexual assault and abuse immediately impacts the 2nd chakra because that is where our sexual organs are located, but it also impacts virtually every other chakra, including the 7th, because it can change the course of our entire lives and life paths; the 6th, because it can cause us to doubt our intuition; the 5th, having to do with self-expression and empowerment; the 4th, having to do with emotions; the 3rd, because it can lead to issues like poor self-esteem, eating disorders, and other addictions; and the 1st chakra, because it can relate to family, trust, security, and safety.

CONDITION SPOTLIGHT

PTSD AND SEXUAL ABUSE AND ASSAULT

PTSD

Post-traumatic stress disorder, or PTSD, is a mental and physical health condition initially brought on by a terrifying event or period of extreme stress, usually defined as trauma. It can last months or even years. Examples of traumatic experiences include sexual assault or abuse, physical or emotional abuse, bullying, being in a serious accident, family conflict, experiences of war, observing violence, or being the victim of a fire or a natural disaster—but this is far from a complete list. Trauma impacts everyone differently, and what is traumatic for one person may not be for someone else. The same is true for PTSD. Depending on the degree of resiliency, underlying mental health conditions, time of exposure, age, available support systems and resources, and other factors, people encountering trauma may or may not develop PTSD. It is normal, nothing to be ashamed of, and definitely not a sign of weakness.

Common symptoms of PTSD include the following:

- Recurrent, unwanted distressing memories of traumatic or very upsetting events
- Reliving the traumatic event as if it were happening again (flashbacks)
- Dreams or nightmares recalling the traumatic event
- Severe emotional or physical reactions to things that remind you of the traumatic event, such as to fireworks if you have been involved in an incident with guns
- Trying to avoid thinking or talking about the traumatic event
- Avoiding places, activities, or people that remind you of the trauma
- Negative thoughts about yourself, other people, or the world after experiencing trauma
- Hopelessness about the future
- Blocking memories related to details of the trauma and how you felt
- Difficulty maintaining close relationships
- Feeling detached from family and friends
- Lack of interest in activities you once enjoyed
- Feeling emotionally numb, having difficulty expressing emotion
- Being easily startled or frightened
- Feeling like you are walking on eggshells, waiting for the next shoe to drop
- Self-destructive behavior, such as drinking too much or driving too fast
- Trouble sleeping and concentrating
- Irritability, angry outbursts, or aggressive behavior
- Overwhelming guilt or shame

Desensitization is another symptom of PTSD, in which people literally feel cut off from their bodies and themselves. Bessel van der Kolk, MD, brilliantly writes about the concept of being desensitized to your feelings in his book *The Body Keeps the Score*, which discusses his work with PTSD patients. The research that he and his colleagues conducted and continue to conduct has shown that even if we are not aware of feelings of fear, rejection, paranoia, helplessness, and other emotions that go along with PTSD, or if we try to deny that we are affected by them, these feelings resonate in our bodies in the form of emotional and physical illness, physical changes in our brains, our "other brains" (our gut), and throughout our bodies.

PTSD victims may not even be conscious of these physical symptoms and likely don't relate them to emotional trauma, because when we lose touch with our feelings, we also lose touch with our bodies and intuition. This is especially common as a result of sexual and physical abuse or assault, since the body is a direct recipient of the trauma. An extreme example of dissociation is multiple personality disorder, or dissociative identity disorder, where parts of a person's identity literally splits off to protect them from the experience and memory of incredibly traumatic events.

I was encouraged to cut myself off from my body and feelings at a young age. I remember being told by my father that I was "making up" feeling carsick every time I rode in the back seat, or that I was "being dramatic." I soon learned to stop talking and took refuge inside of myself.

Years before the eating disorder behaviors began, I had the traumatic experience of being bullied. My period arrived a month before my eleventh birthday. Having it come at such a young age was an experience that I soon came to resent rather than rejoice in. An early period meant breasts forming at an age when I still thought of myself as a child, hair on my arms and legs while everyone around me was mostly still smooth and near-hairless; for me it was an early start to one of life's biggest changes, which I was completely unprepared for. Many people wouldn't think of breasts as being inherently unpleasant, but for a ten-year-old girl it's much easier and safer to be flat-chested like all the other little girls. I can remember being gawked at on the street by older boys and men. It was embarrassing and disgusting to be leered at.

Perhaps because I was well-endowed, when I was in fifth grade, my mom decided that menstruation was imminent. She gave me a feminine pad to keep in my pocketbook, even though I hadn't had my first period. Another girl in my class saw it when we were in the bathroom together and asked if I got my period. I said no, which was the truth, but she didn't believe me. She and another girl, who was equally well-developed and had clearly reached puberty, decided to tell the rest of our group of "friends." They began a daily ritual of making me feel as bad as they possibly could. We were in every class together. I lived in a small town with only one middle school, so I felt trapped. The bullying lasted from April until the end of the school year, when they informed me they wouldn't torment me the next year. It wasn't just teasing about getting my period—it was also about having breasts, getting a zit, or not liking my hair that day. They would use anything they could find or invent to tear me down. They were classic bullies who behaved like a pack of jackals gathered around a frightened animal.

Looking back, I can see that they were also normal fifth-grade girls, at least normal within a culture that teaches women to compete like wolves for an alpha position. Countless people, both men and women, have experienced this kind of traumatic treatment as children.

I felt so ashamed that I didn't tell my parents anything, thinking of myself as a loser for not knowing how to fix this. I became depressed and withdrawn, different from my usually rapid talking and rather hyper self. Bullying, at a time when my body and self-image were transforming rapidly, is one of the events I can link to my eating disorder. In the aftermath, I dealt with a range of negative repercussions—hating my body, shame, wondering if it was my fault, not being able to tell anyone, feeling powerless, rejection of my female characteristics and sexualtiy, a lack of ability to trust, and more. These feelings are classic reactions to trauma, whether it be the all-too-common experience of being bullied or other forms of trauma like sexual abuse.

I have come to terms with all of this and still talk to some of the people involved in these incidents. They long ago apologized and I long ago forgave them. This time shaped so much of my life for years to come, and no doubt similar experiences have shaped the lives of other young people, so I hope that by telling my story, I can help others heal.

Sexual Abuse and Assault

The psychological or behavioral effects of someone who has been sexually abused or assaulted can include the following:[4]

- Feeling separated from your body or yourself
- Trusting too easily or not trusting at all
- Difficulty setting or recognizing boundaries, since yours were violated and ignored
- Obsessive thoughts recalling the abuse
- Self-medicating with drugs, alcohol, or other things to try to push down feelings
- Low self-esteem
- Trouble with intimacy
- Sexual promiscuity
- Suicidal thoughts, attempts, and self-harm
- Eating disorders, body-image issues
- Sexual dysfunction/lack of pleasure
- Anxiety, depression, panic attacks

- Possible abuse of others
- Difficulty concentrating
- Fear of medical procedures

The emotional effects can include:

- Grief over lost childhood experiences
- Guilt and confusion regarding possible physical pleasure during the abuse
- Shame, both from "allowing" the victimization and not being able to tell anyone
- Anger and rage, sometimes out of nowhere

The physical effects can include:

- Gastrointestinal issues and pelvic pain
- Headaches
- Back pain
- Pain during sex
- Increased frequency of obesity
- Intense gag reflex

I frequently encounter people with physical issues, like fibroids, endometriosis, sexual dysfunction, difficult menstrual cycles, cystitis, polycystic ovary syndrome, and cancer in the reproductive organs, who have been sexually abused or assaulted, especially people who have not begun the healing process. These issues can also be linked to an inability to express feminine or masculine power due to possible shame or bullying that was experienced in relation to sexual identity. I often pick up energy in the 2nd chakra that is angry, trapped, swirling around in circles, and ashamed. This type of "negative" energy contributes to unhealthy cell growth, uterine and intestinal cramping, inflammation, and other diseases. Refer back to chapter 5 for some suggestions on how to release negative energy.

I have worked with survivors of PTSD, including from sexual abuse and assault, of all ages, for the past thirty years. I've learned that a common cause of lasting trauma is the intense fear that the abuse, or something similar, will happen again, along with feeling powerless to stop or prevent it. It is incredibly important to remember that you have been through the worst and that you are a different, stronger person. The conditions, like age or maturity, for example, that may have put you at risk of being a victim, are not present anymore. Even if you were once not believed or supported, it's essential to reach out to someone you trust, perhaps a trained professional, and talk about what happened.

Strategies for Healing from PTSD and Sexual Abuse and Assault

- If you haven't already, tell your story to a trusted friend, family member, or therapist. Unfortunately, trauma, including sexual abuse and assault are not uncommon. According to the advocacy website for RAINN (Rape, Abuse & Incest National Network),[5] one in six people in America have survived rape or attempted rape. Every seventy-three seconds, someone is sexually assaulted, but only five out of a thousand offenders end up in prison. Transgender individuals are even more at risk, at a frequency of 21 percent, versus 18 percent of non-transgender females and 4 percent of non-transgender males being the victims of sexual assault or attempts. You are not alone, and it is important to receive support and validation, even if your attempts to tell someone what happened to you in the past have been met with less-than-positive reactions.

- EMDR, or eye movement desensitization and reprocessing, is a therapeutic technique in which participants recall traumatic events and their feelings. This is a systematic process, done at the survivor's pace and comfort level. It includes directed eye movements, tapping, and audio stimulation, which help retrieve and release physical and emotional symptoms and impact at the time of the traumatic events. This is a professionally recognized procedure, usually paid for by insurance. I personally found it to be very helpful.

- Work on self-love and self-acceptance, especially if you are dealing with confusing and conflicting feelings and memories. Also work on connecting with and listening to your intuition. During childhood abuse, especially, the victimizer uses psychological "tricks" to tell the victim that what is happening is okay, normal, fun—and often their fault. They teach victims to ignore and push down their feelings and intuition, which can result in the loss of a personal identity. I would especially recommend a therapist trained in Jungian psychology and also someone trained in cognitive behavioral therapy, which works on challenging and changing unhelpful and false beliefs and behaviors and teaching healthy coping mechanisms when faced with stress or trauma.

- Dance and other movement can be great for connecting with the body in loving and nurturing ways, reversing the learned behavior of disconnection with the body during the abuse or assault. Strength training with weights or using resistance from your body helps you to know that you can better defend yourself in the future and has the side effect of increased emotional strength and empowerment as well.

- Find a form of stress relief you love and make it a regular practice. Anxiety, depression, anger, and grief build up in the body in the form of negative energy. As I have discussed, this type of energy needs to be released, physically, in order to prevent physical and emotional symptoms and heal the symptoms currently present. Stress relief, whether it is in the form of creativity, meditation, being in nature, talking to friends, movement, or watching funny movies is also an excellent distraction and breaks the stream of thoughts many of us find as constant companions, whether we have been the victim of trauma or not.

- Education and advocacy work, such as volunteering with charities that assist victims of abuse can be both empowering and therapeutic for survivors. However, it can also be triggering or be used as a way to avoid dealing with one's own grief and trauma. Once you have processed your personal experience and are well on the way to healing, I strongly encourage it.

These are just a few suggestions that my clients and I have found to be helpful when healing from trauma.

CASE STUDY

Jill, age thirty-two, contacted me for assistance with trauma, including prolonged sexual abuse and anxiety.

2ND CHAKRA ISSUES

- Very sensitive
- Difficulty expressing herself
- Survivor of prolonged sexual abuse
- Gut issues
- Self-esteem issues but very strong-willed and professionally accomplished
- Body image issues, frequent thoughts about weight, calories, and food
- Adrenal fatigue, always "on"
- Dysfunctional family
- Shame

OTHER CHAKRA ISSUES/STRENGTHS

- Spiritual awakening (7th)
- Anxiety (6th)
- Very empathic (4th)
- Need to let go of the past (1st)
- Had to take care of herself from a young age (1st)
- Need for control (4th)
- Sensitive to toxins, mold exposure (6th)

When I shared what my guides had told me, Jill said it was like I had known her my entire life. She contacted me because she had recently told her mother about being the victim of sexual abuse, incest. She was abused by her father from ages six to fourteen and had never told anyone except her mother and her husband, and not until very recently. She had held in the shame, pain, and fear for the majority of her life. As·is often the case, the fact that my guides already knew about the abuse and revealed it in the report made it easier for her to talk about it with me.

Her father was a very prominent man in the community, and she was afraid that if she said anything, she would not be believed. She was also sure he had likely abused others, even possibly other members of her family. He had passed away, which was why she finally felt safe telling someone. Her mother said that she was not aware of the abuse but had divorced him and remarried when Jill was in her early teens.

Jill is one of the strongest women I have ever met. One would expect that she wouldn't be able to function, that she would struggle deeply with mental health, addiction, or have difficulty maintaining relationships, but she is highly intelligent, with an excellent job, and takes very good care of herself. She wanted to work on boundaries, which she had never learned, and on moving forward from the trauma of the past so that she could be the best mom for her children.

We began working together weekly, exploring the ways that her physical symptoms, like gut issues, fatigue, and anxiety, might be manifestations of the trauma she had to push down for so many years. We worked on connection to intuition and her body, which she had never been taught to trust, and on accepting and loving herself, unconditionally. I provided a safe space to talk about the confusing love she felt for her father, her fear and hatred of him, and the helplessness she felt until she was able to put a stop to the abuse at the age of fourteen. We also worked on helping her identify areas in her life where she tried to exert control as a coping mechanism for feeling insecure and anxious, such as sometimes obsessive thinking about weight, food, and calories. Instead we substituted healthy coping mechanisms that increased confidence and reduced anxiety—like making time for regular exercise, time in nature, and creative activities with her kids. She was receptive to my suggestion that she try a pole fitness class when she expressed interest in the classes I take. It often helps people to feel attractive, desirable, and even sexy in a safe, controlled environment with other supportive people.

I also recommended supplements, food, and strategies to support her adrenals, emotional health, and gut health. Over our months together, we peeled back the onion layers, and eventually our visits became monthly and bimonthly, rather than weekly. Her emotional, physical, and spiritual health has flourished, and I am extremely blessed and privileged to have seen her heal and grow before my eyes.

END OF CHAPTER 13 QUESTIONS

1. How has trauma impacted you? What emotions do you associate with this impact?
2. Has the impact changed over time?

3. What parts of this chapter most resonated with you?
4. What are your spiritual and emotional symptoms associated with issues you may have in the 2nd chakra?
5. If you have received help for dealing with trauma, what aspects have been most and least helpful?
6. Which current life situations are influencing the symptoms you are having associated with the 2nd chakra?
7. Which situations in your early life are influencing the symptoms you are having associated with the 2nd chakra?

14

Trust, Safety, Security, and Family

Healing Using the 1st Chakra

The greatest burden a child must bear is the unlived life of
the parents.

—Carl Jung

Overall themes: safety, security, trust,
basic needs, and family

1ST CHAKRA

The 1st chakra is also called the root chakra and is symbolized by the color red. It is located at the base of the spine. The
Sanskrit name for the 1st chakra is *Maladhara,* meaning "root
support." Root chakra issues are some of the most important
to address because the root chakra is the base of safety, security, and basic needs. If we do not have a safe place to live, food
to eat, money to live on, and a healthy, supportive family, it is
very difficult to address other issues in our lives. Without these
basic necessities, we live in a state of constant anxiety. There is
no time for creativity, spiritual growth, or thoughts of higher
life purpose.

Location	Physical Issues	Emotional and Spiritual Concerns
Base of spine Blood Joints, muscles Immune system Lymphatic system Skin Rectum	Blood diseases Autoimmune disorders Immune deficiency AIDS Broken bones, bone density Joint inflammation Muscle weakness and pain Skin cancer, sensitivity, rashes General inflammation Varicose veins Sciatica Lower spine	Family issues, including dysfunctional family Substance abuse, mental illness, trauma in family or family history Trust, safety, basic needs Caretaking Support systems and belonging Healthy boundaries

POSSIBLE PHYSICAL, EMOTIONAL, AND SPIRITUAL ROOT CAUSES FOR ISSUES IN THIS CHAKRA

- Addiction in family, family dysfunction
- Viruses
- Being a caretaker
- Lack of proper boundary setting or having boundaries respected
- Improper nutrition or difficulty absorbing nutrients
- Autoimmune disease
- Conditions impacting the blood
- Low bone density
- Scoliosis or other spinal conditions
- Skin conditions
- Circulation issues

INTUITIVE WRITING PROMPTS

- What could I do to feel emotionally safer? Was there ever a time when I felt safe?
- What impact did my role models have on this chakra?
- How can I create change and break the cycle of dysfunction? How have I already done this?

CALL TO ACTION

If you are having symptoms in this chakra, I believe that your intuition and Spirit are calling on you to work on the following if you want to attain physical, emotional, and spiritual health.

PHYSICAL

1. Learn about family history of autoimmune disease, which can include diabetes, heart disease, and many skin conditions.
2. Eat in an anti-inflammatory manner, avoiding sugar, alcohol, processed foods, gluten, and dairy, and make most of your diet plant-based.
3. Address spinal and neck alignment, conditions that impact the spine. Be sure to stretch and move your back frequently to avoid disc degeneration and stiffness.
4. Get tested for ferritin (iron storage) and iron levels. Address possible issues of iron absorption and diseases impacting storage of iron, like hemochromatosis.
5. Address varicose veins, which can cause pain and fatigue.
6. Get tested for bone density and take measures to protect the health of your bones starting at an early age. Testing is normally recommended for people fifty and above, unless symptoms occur earlier.

7. After receiving vaccines, take measures with a natural practitioner to detox afterward, and try not to get multiple vaccines at the same time.

EMOTIONAL

1. Get support for healing family dysfunction issues, including addiction, so that you can break the cycle.
2. Work on identifying and healing trauma and releasing outdated, negative messages you have heard from others and have told yourself.
3. Balance your caretaking responsibilities with self-care.
4. Address issues around trust and safety.

AFFIRMATIONS AND VISUALIZATIONS FOR THE 1ST CHAKRA

Affirmations:

- I have everything I need.
- I am never alone.
- I can set healthy boundaries.
- I am grounded and safe.
- I can live in the present and let the past go.
- It's okay to be different from my family.
- I send myself love and acceptance.

Visualizations:

- Imagine saying no and setting boundaries with family and friends.
- Feel yourself being supported and loved unconditionally.
- Visualize being filled with strength and inspiring others with that strength.

CONDITION SPOTLIGHT

DYSFUNCTIONAL AND ALCOHOLIC FAMILIES

Naturally, the family systems that you and your parents came from will influence your personality, your health, your spirituality, your relationships—virtually every aspect of your life. For this reason, I often pick up information about family members, both alive and passed, as well as family history in the 1st chakra part of my readings.

An important part of 1st chakra health is feeling emotionally and physically safe. It's difficult to feel that way in a dysfunctional family, in which the people who are supposed to be loving and caring for you are not doing that because of mental illness, addiction, or narcissism. Growing up in poverty also makes safety and security difficult. Parents often have to work two or three jobs just to get by and may be forced to house their families in high-crime areas with lower quality schools. Single parenthood amplifies these issues even more.

Issues related to childhood are the root causes or contribute to the root causes of the majority of problems clients come to me with, in every chakra. They are most commonly related to dysfunctional family issues in the past and present, but they can also relate to bullying, childhood illness and accidents, grief from losing a loved one, and having psychic or empathic experiences a person may have been too young to understand.

Intergenerational dysfunction is especially problematic because the unhealthy behaviors and thoughts have often been normalized as they are passed from generation to generation, including possibly influencing DNA through epigenetics. Our genetic inheritance is not strictly limited to the content of the DNA sequence we've inherited from our parents. Chemical compounds that are added to single genes can regulate their activity and affect how the gene is expressed; these modifications are known as epigenetic changes. The epigenome comprises all of the chemical compounds that have been added to the entirety of one's DNA (genome) as a way to regulate the activity (expression) of all the genes within the genome. The chemical compounds of the epigenome are not part of the DNA sequence, but are on or attached to DNA (*epi* means "above" in Greek). Epigenetic modifications remain as cells divide, and in some cases can be inherited through the generations. Environmental influences, such as a person's diet and exposure to pollutants, can also impact the epigenome.[6]

Studies have been conducted showing that trauma, stress, and other emotional factors create epigenetic changes in mice.[7] The jury is still out regarding how it works in humans, but I have received information from my guides that not only can emotional experiences influence the genome, but conversely, therapy, healing work, and recovery can reverse negative epigenetic changes that took place in earlier generations. This potentially has enormous implications.

The development of mental illness is not guaranteed by genetic propensity. It has long been known that by providing a healthy, loving, supportive environment for children, they are far less likely to develop things like anxiety, depression, bipolar disorder, and schizophrenia, even if they possess the genes for it. It is also widely known that childhood trauma greatly increases the risk for developing these issues.

If our emotional experiences do indeed influence genetic expression, this means that by getting help for mental illness, healing from trauma, and removing ourselves from the negative energy and behavior of family and friends, we can not only positively change our own genetic makeup but also lessen the chance that mental illness, addiction, and neurological disorders will be passed on to our children and our children's children. We can truly break the cycle of pain and dysfunction and help future generations avoid the 1st chakra issues I have discussed. The following story from my family illustrates how insidious and destructive untreated generational trauma can be.

Black Sheep Santa

Like all good Italians, my father's side of the family spent every Christmas Eve celebrating a tradition called *La Vigilia*, or the Feast of the Seven Fishes. We packed my grandmother's house in Connecticut, at least seven families plus guests. Everyone looked forward to it. Each year a different uncle, or sometimes my grandfather, would get dressed up and play Santa, handing out the presents purchased by my grandmother to all of the grandchildren.

One Christmas, when I was about ten years old, a few of my cousins and I started searching under the tree to find the presents with our names on them. As I searched, I noticed that neither my nor my brothers' names were on any of the presents. I didn't say anything to my cousins.

I remember telling my mother, and I can still see the look on her face. Her eyes and lips fell wide open. "Are you sure?" she said. We both looked under the tree and she couldn't find presents with our names on them, either. She told my father, and he looked more angry than surprised. He had a great deal of animosity toward my grandmother for how he said she had treated him most of his life.

My parents left the house immediately and headed for Toys "R" Us, only about fifteen minutes away, thankfully still open on Christmas Eve. I met my mom at the door of the living room in the back of the house when they returned, smuggling Christmas presents under the tree before my younger brothers could realize something was wrong.

As my father came through the door dressed as Santa, his jet-black hair peeking out from under the white fluffy wig, I watched for my grandmother's reaction as he called my brothers' and my names again and again, handing us large, brightly colored presents from under the tree. I studied her first shocked, then angry, then terrified face, picking up her energy. Aside from the fear of realizing that my parents had figured out what she had done, anticipating the later confrontation and other ramifications, she felt cold. She always felt cold to me. Her eyes were lifeless and dull, her lips pursed tightly together in the familiar puss I often noticed. I always felt the evil in her, even from a very young age.

Sadly, none of my aunts or uncles seemed to care about what my grandmother had done to us. I heard my parents tell them that night and several other times at later dates but they made excuses for her. Perhaps they were afraid of incurring her wrath themselves, but I think they were just cowards. My grandmother picked and chose which children she treated well and which she seemed to emotionally abuse, which I observed myself on repeated occasions. She created the perfect petri dish for systemic family dysfunction.

Adult Children of Alcoholics

Even though I did not come from an alcoholic family, I found valuable help from a group devoted to helping people who have. Adult Children of Alcoholics, or ACOA,[8] is a twelve-step support program to help people raised in dysfunctional families of all sorts. More information can be found on their website, including a list of characteristics. Many people raised in dysfunctional families experience the following:

1. Isolation and fear of authority figures
2. Seeking approval that results in a loss of true self; difficulty feeling and expressing these feelings
3. Fear of angry people and being overly sensitive to criticism
4. Tendency to become addicted and/or marry people with characteristics and behaviors similar to our parents
5. Fear of abandonment
6. Relating to life as a victim and seeking out other similar personalities we can save; may confuse caretaking/saving with love, also called codependency

7. Living to take care of others rather than looking inward at ourselves and our own issues
8. Difficulty establishing healthy boundaries, feeling fearful or guilty when we express our needs and opinions
9. Addiction to adrenaline and excitement; may choose careers that reflect this, such as the helping professions, high-risk jobs
10. Low self-esteem, perfectionism, and self-esteem tied to performance, appearance, weight
11. Difficulty coping with stress, anger, and loss; not having learned appropriate coping strategies or ways to express healthy emotions from our parents

A key task for a person raised in a dysfunctional home is individuation: becoming a separate entity, with feelings, beliefs, and behaviors determined by one's own intuition and life, rather than being impacted by the feelings, beliefs, and behaviors of others. It's about learning to love and accept yourself unconditionally, without the burden of outside judgment. That is not to say that there are not things we may want and need to change, or that we never pay attention to the observations and opinions of others, especially people we care about or who care about us. Of course we do, but we must not make others our central focus.

I have observed with clients, as well as in my own family, that there are often "identified patients" who take on the burden of being the "truth teller" and symptom holder for everyone else. This is different from being the parent or parents with the addiction, mental illness, or other disorder. Sadly, the parent(s)' problems are usually denied and go untreated, which is the cause of the family dysfunction. The "identified patient" is the child or children who understands that the parent(s)' behavior is creating problems and who may try to talk about it but is ignored or faced with rejection. They may be told that they are "crazy." They usually take the brunt of the abandonment or abuse, effectively taking the attention away from the parent(s) and central problematic issues.

It is not uncommon for these children to develop eating disorders, addictions, or have problems with the law or in school, which also defers attention away from the core family issues. I was one of the people who played that role in my family. Sometimes, the identified patients end up becoming the emotionally and spiritually healthiest members of the family, if they receive therapy that teaches them to express and address their feelings. If they are fortunate and strong enough, they get help and move past the family dysfunction, sometimes assisting the family system in getting help as well.

In addition to the identified patient, these are some other common roles found in dysfunctional families:

- The "peacemaker," who always tries to avoid and quell conflict
- The "truth teller," who exposes denial and confronts family members about their behavior
- The "black sheep," the one who doesn't quite fit in and who everyone blames for their unhappiness

It can be a tough road for the children in dysfunctional families who stand up for themselves and dare to expose the family secrets and issues that the rest of the family is so invested in hiding and pretending don't exist. It was for me. I don't fit in and can't relate to the people I grew up with, but looking back, I never felt like I did. The good news is that we find people we can relate to, who love and accept us in ways we never experienced from the people who should have. We make our own families with friends, and we create our own new families, raising our children and conducting our relationships in healthy ways.

Strategies for Dealing with Dysfunctional Family Situations and Breaking the Cycle

- Try not to take the behavior of others personally. Even if you have been blamed for someone else's bad behavior, which often happens in the case of narcissistic people who cannot look inward, know that it is never the fault of a child who is mistreated. We cannot change the thoughts or behavior of others, only our own.

- Allow your feelings of hurt, abandonment, anger, and other pain, even and especially if you are afraid of them. You have already been through the worst and have survived. Only by letting the emotions surface can they be released.

- Forgiveness is an important tool, primarily for you. I love the saying about taking poison but wishing someone else will die. Anger is one of the most powerful poisons, capable of inflicting long-term emotional, physical, and spiritual damage. It doesn't mean that you are excusing bad or hurtful behavior, just that you want to release it, and the person who inflicted it, from your life.

- Depersonalize the hurtful behavior. This has been a helpful strategy for me. While addiction is a component of the dysfunction in our family, substance abuse is not, but I use this analogy to think of the people who have hurt me as a bottle of alcohol. Addicted people are constantly in an altered state and not operating as their authentic selves. Since addiction is a progressive disease, they often have missed important developmental stages of maturity and are not capable of behaving or thinking the same way as someone who has not been impacted by addiction. It is the same for mental illness.

- It's impossible to talk with an inanimate object, like a bottle, which is why it is so frustrating and hurtful to try to talk with an addicted person. How many times have you talked to, yelled at, or pleaded with a dysfunctional family member or friend, only to have it be a waste of time? That isn't your fault. There are some people who will never be able to hear you and respond the way you need them to.

- Decide what you want and need from your important relationships and evaluate whether that is possible. I have worked with people who for literally their entire lives, sometimes forty, fifty, or even sixty years, have been grieving the kind of family they wished they could have had. They never stopped trying to change the thoughts and behaviors of people who have hurt them and still base their self-esteem on what these same people say and do.

- Be aware of relating to your parents or siblings the way you did when you were a child. It is possible that your emotional and spiritual growth has been stunted, and that you have never developed a true, separate relationship with yourself. You may be still living in the past, blocked by fear and grief from moving on. Sometimes we just need to accept that things didn't turn out the way we wanted.

- Take control of difficult relationships and set healthy boundaries. Turn off your phone or don't answer it when people who make you feel bad call or text. You don't owe them a response. Block people from social media, as many times as you need to—even if you have relatives, like mine, who create fake accounts so that they can still harass and stalk you. If you don't know how to make your social media accounts private, ask someone who does. Limit what you post if you choose to participate in social media. Your business should stay your business. If you have people who show up at your home or place of business unannounced, do not be afraid to tell them that you are busy, even if you have to physically leave to get the point across. Say no if you do not want to visit, even if you feel obligated. You will end up resenting yourself if you don't. It is also okay if you need to remove yourself from relationships and cut off contact. Family members who treat you badly are not acting like true family. Setting healthy boundaries also models doing the same for your children.

- My husband and I firmly believe that we raised healthy, happy, successful children because we learned from how we were brought up and didn't make the same mistakes. How you raise your kids is your business, not anyone else's. Don't be afraid to tell others to butt out.

- Make your mental health and the health of your family a priority. Take care of your problematic issues before they impact the people you love or as soon as you notice that they might. Seek out help from therapists and educate yourself about the ways growing up in a dysfunctional family may have impacted you. Self-help groups like Adult Children of Alcoholics are great resources.

CASE STUDY

The following case study is about a woman, Sheila, age twenty-nine, with autoimmune illness. Trauma related to dealing with dysfunctional family members was one of the root causes.

1ST CHAKRA ISSUES

- Immune system weakness
- Autoimmune symptoms, including those similar to Lyme disease and Lyme coinfections
- Weakness and tingling in arms and legs, fingers
- Lack of trust in people and the universe, trouble setting boundaries (and 2nd and 6th)
- Dysfunctional family of origin
- Dysfunctional marriage (and 2nd)

OTHER CHAKRA ISSUES

- Chronic illness (7th)
- Migraine headaches (6th)
- Gut inflammation, irregularities, sensitivities (3rd)
- Highly sensitive to chemicals (6th)
- Highly sensitive to others, empathic (4th)
- Fear of connecting to intuition and authentic self (6th, 3rd)
- Tendency to isolate (2nd)
- Need for control (4th)

The painting I created for Sheila showed the green curlicue lines that often symbolize Lyme disease and virus-related issues for me, as well as blue in the gut area, signifying someone who picks up the emotions of herself and others in her gut and who may have related symptoms. I painted magenta around her heart and throat chakra areas, which was a sign to me that she desperately needed to express her authentic self.

When we went over the report and painting together, I learned that she had been diagnosed with Lyme disease, several coinfections, and an underlying chronic fatigue virus approximately three years before. After initially finding some improvement through traditional treatments, she hadn't made any progress toward healing in the past two and half years.

Some days she had trouble getting out of bed. Specialists were of no help, and other traditional treatments had actually made her symptoms worse. She felt completely helpless and often hopeless, but there was still part of her who thought that recovery was possible, she just didn't know how to get there.

Understandably, she had spent hours each day for years on the internet and social media, doing research into possible treatments, practitioners, root causes, people who have recovered—literally anything she could get her hands on. She identified herself on social media as a "Lyme Warrior," complete with a green glow around her photo, often signifying Lyme disease.

In her case, the root causes of her illness included mold exposure in the past, which had triggered her Lyme disease symptoms to appear (she did not remember a tick bite), needing to stand up for herself and leave a marriage that she hadn't been happy in since it started, and needing to be in a profession that involved creativity and spirituality, rather than customer service, which she hated. She also needed to emotionally separate and set appropriate boundaries with her father, who was an abusive alcoholic. Over time, we worked on these issues together. I referred her to a specialist I commonly work with and made recommendations about diet, movement, meditation, communication with intuition, and more.

I wanted to be sure to address the intense anxiety she felt on a daily basis, which I believed was being contributed to by her continuous focus on her illness and on being a patient. That was her entire identity. She shared that she was terrified to take her mind off her illness because she thought she would be "dropping the ball" and somehow not be focused on healing. She was convinced that if she let go of control and allowed God, Spirit, or the universe to take care of her, that she would become sicker or not heal. This is a very common phenomenon I have encountered.

I shared with her that when I found out I had Lyme disease and a host of related issues, I was, of course, afraid, and my first impulse was to let anxiety take over. But I knew that anxiety would only slow my healing. As I worked toward healing, I refused to take ownership of my illness, never letting it define my identity or personality. I actively told myself things like "you are healthy"; "you are strong and capable"; "you are healing"; "trust your intuition"; "you are safe and being taken care of." When I did, I could feel my anxiety decrease and my optimism rise.

I wasn't in denial, in fact, quite the opposite. I was promoting healing. I didn't let "being sick" get in the way of having fun, spending time with my family and friends, and attending to my responsibilities. I rested when my body told me to, ate an extremely healthy anti-inflammatory diet because it made me feel better, and followed all of my doctor's advice about detoxing, using the remedies and doing the treatments, believing that they would heal me completely. I suggested that Sheila try a similar approach in her own healing.

At first, Sheila thought that by my suggesting she try this, I was diminishing her illness and symptoms. But the more we talked about how labels can be useful as well as anxiety provoking and limiting, the more she understood that the way she had been living her life wasn't working. It was worth trying a different way.

She feared that people wouldn't want to spend time with "a sick person," so she hadn't been reaching out, but she was wrong. Her friends and family cared very much and enjoyed her company, but they felt helpless. She thought that spending just half an hour or hour on creative activities, because that is all she had the energy for, was a waste of time. But once she allowed herself to enjoy writing, putting together puzzles, and creating small terrariums again, she realized how much she had been missing this aspect of herself. Not only was it a wonderful diversion from thinking about not feeling well, she felt like she was accomplishing something, and it did wonders for her self-esteem. She had other labels to add to her identity, like "person who faces her fears," "creative person," "photographer," "plant lover," etc.

As Sheila took these steps, she began to not only get her life back, but to create an entirely new one, with interests and a more outgoing nature she would not otherwise have had. In approximately six months, she was consistently out of bed, and while not completely free of symptoms, she was well on her way. A year later, she was symptom-free the majority of the time and headed toward a complete recovery.

END OF CHAPTER 14 QUESTIONS

1. Has family dysfunction impacted you? If so, how?
2. How have you worked to break the cycle of family dysfunction? What fears and beliefs are holding you back?
3. Are you able to set healthy boundaries and express your feelings with family members? If not, how is this impacting your life?
4. What did you feel were the most important parts of this chapter for you? What are your takeaways?
5. What role have you taken on in your family? Common roles are the peacemaker, the truth teller, the identified patient, and the black sheep.
6. Are you more emotionally, healthy, and spiritually evolved than other members of your family? What issues and feelings has this created for you?
7. Have you had to cut off contact with toxic family members? Are you feeling guilty about that, or are you at peace with your decision?
8. What are your spiritual and emotional symptoms associated with issues you may have in the 1st chakra?

PART II

Glossary of Healing

Even if you have a terminal disease, you don't have to sit down and mope. Enjoy life and challenge the illness that you have.

—Nelson Mandela

This glossary contains information about root causes and treatment for individual issues, listed alphabetically. For further guidance, you can also refer to the general Call to Action items near the end of chapter 7, and the more specific Call to Action items found in each chakra chapter.

In this section, I make suggestions for supplements, herbs, and vitamins that might be helpful, but I highly recommend using them only under the care and recommendation of a health-care professional. Self-medicating, even with natural supplements, can be dangerous and can worsen symptoms. The doses and combinations should be determined by a professional specifically for you and monitored so that if you have any side effects, the culprit can be identified and discontinued or the dose modified. It is always best to try to obtain nutrients from food, rather than supplements, if possible, which aids absorption and reduces the possibility of side effects.

If you are not able to work with a health-care professional, please do extensive research before beginning any supplement, including possible side effects, reactions with medications and other supplements, and doses and options for the form (liquid, skin patch, pill, etc.). Start with a very low dose and add only one new thing at a time, so that if side effects occur, you will know the culprit.

Educate yourself about the active ingredient(s) in the supplement as well. For instance, curcumin is the active ingredient in turmeric, and DHA and EPA are the active ingredients in omega-3s. Labels can be very deceiving. A dose of 500 mg of turmeric will not have the same results as 500 mg of curcumin, for example. Often the price of some supplements can be lower because they don't contain as much of the active ingredient, so price does matter. Pay attention to where the ingredients were sourced and to the fillers. You want supplements to be as pure as possible. The ingredients should be grown and produced in countries that have strict standards for safety and pesticide use.

ACID REFLUX AND BARRETT'S ESOPHAGUS
Chakras 5, 3

Acid reflux (also called GERD or gastroesophageal reflux disease in its chronic form) is a common condition that can seriously impact quality of life, not only because of pain and discomfort but also by interfering with sleep and the ability to attend social functions or go out to dinner. Physical root causes include side effects of medication like anti-inflammatories, nitrates, alpha-blockers, sedatives, and antibiotics; hiatial hernia (when part of the stomach protrudes through the diaphragm); pregnancy; smoking; and being overweight. Taking medication for acid reflux often relieves the symptoms but does not address the root causes and can make the situation worse, especially since these conditions are often caused by inadequate production of stomach acid, not an excess. Antacids are one of the first recommendations doctors suggest and one of the first "remedies" people try over the counter, since they are so readily available and are generally considered safe. This class of medications is not without side effects, however, which include the following:

- Acid *rebound*, which is when the stomach produces even more acid than before starting the medication
- Milk-alkali syndrome, causing possible symptoms of headache, nausea, irritability, weakness, high blood-calcium levels, and reduced kidney function
- Hypophosphatemia (low phosphate levels in the blood), from high doses of aluminum containing antacids, which could lead to muscle weakness, anorexia, and softening of the bones
- Potential danger for people who have high blood pressure, chronic heart or renal failure, and others who have sodium restricted diets, since some antacids are sodium based

I have worked with many people who have this common condition and found that the use of a general digestive enzyme, probiotics, and dietary modification can solve the problems permanently, without the need for medication. Pay attention to when acid reflux occurs and what you have consumed. Stress reduction is also very important.

Barrett's Esophagus is a change in the lining of the esophagus, thought to be caused by prolonged acid reflux, but I know people who have it who do not have acid reflux. It is not dangerous in itself, but could possibly be a precursor to esophageal cancer. As with a hiatial hernia, sometimes surgery is required when other measures have not been successful.

Getting adequate fiber has been shown to be helpful. Foods to avoid with these conditions include:

- Alcohol
- Sugar and processed carbs
- Coffee
- Tea
- Milk and dairy
- Chocolate
- Peppermint
- Tomatoes, tomato sauce, and ketchup
- French fries
- Battered fish
- Tempura
- Onion rings
- Red meat
- Processed meats
- Mustard
- Spicy foods

Spiritually, pay attention to feelings and thoughts you have that you have not allowed to come to the surface, and to thoughts that may be playing over and over again in your mind. This "regurgitation" may be physically playing out in your stomach and esophagus. I have found that anger, feeling victimized, and feeling helpless are common feelings that people with acid reflux and related disorders are struggling with.

ADD AND ADHD
Chakras 6, 3, 2

The difference between ADD and ADHD is that ADHD includes "hyperactivity" as a symptom. Usually this is the easier to diagnose of the two because this hyperactivity is often a problem in school settings where children are expected to sit still. Sadly, many children are misdiagnosed with these disorders because their learning styles and energy levels are not a good fit for traditional education, which includes very little time for stress release and physical exercise.

The symptoms of ADD and ADHD are not exclusive to these disorders; in fact, they are common to many other diagnoses and positive traits, like being highly creative and highly intelligent, along with anxiety, depression, neurological disorders, autism and Asperger's syndrome, bipolar disorder, and more. Multiple diagnoses are common, and it isn't necessarily as important to assign labels as it is to help people feel better and function at higher levels. The symptoms of ADD and ADHD include the following:

- Impulsivity
- Anxiety
- Difficulty focusing and paying attention
- Aggression
- Irritability
- Being easily bored
- Quick mood swings
- Difficulty multitasking
- Hyperfocus
- Difficulty with time management and organization
- Trouble finishing tasks
- Emotional sensitivity
- Trouble forming relationships

Traditionally, ADD and ADHD have been treated with stimulant drugs and sometimes therapy, but these drugs can have serious side effects, especially for children, and are addictive.

Their effectiveness is limited, and sometimes they are not effective at all.

Natural remedies I have found to be effective for ADD and ADHD symptoms include:

- Exercise
- Becoming involved in creative projects
- Getting organized
- Counseling
- Acupuncture
- Eating a healthy diet, including omega-3s, complete proteins, and B vitamins, and avoiding sugar and processed foods
- Eating protein and/or fat when consuming carbohydrates or caffeine can help maintain steady levels of blood sugar
- Adequate sleep
- Meditation, especially mindfulness
- Avoid toxins in food, the environment, and in personal products

In addition to the remedies I have listed, it is important to identify and treat possible underlying conditions for ADHD symptoms. These include anxiety, depression, nutritional issues such as malabsorption from gut issues and genetic conditions, thyroid disorders (both hyper and hypo), mold toxicity, Lyme disease, and medication side effects.

As a mental health counselor for over thirty years, much of this time with children, I have found that it is helpful to focus on problem-solving difficult behaviors, rather than making people feel like there is something "wrong" with them. If someone is having difficulty paying attention, perhaps the information they are exposed to is boring or unchallenging. Irritability, becoming easily frustrated, and mood swings can happen because of trauma and justified anger. Emotional sensitivity and difficulty with relationships can happen when people are empaths or when healthy relationships and coping skills haven't been modeled. Many of these symptoms can occur when a person has been raised in a dysfunctional home setting and with addiction. Under these circumstances, a person with true neurological ADD or ADHD would exhibit these symptoms more severely, but none of this means that medication is necessary. It is also important to note that highly intelligent and creative people may be more likely to be misdiagnosed.

Spiritually, if you are having difficulty paying attention, it may be that you do not want to or cannot handle situations or people in your life. Also, your intuition and Spirit may be protecting you from remembering traumatic experiences.

ADDICTION
Chakras 3, 4, 5

Addiction is a way to stop thinking and feeling, but it doesn't work. It only creates larger and more complex problems. People can literally be addicted to anything, along with the usual suspects of gambling, drugs, food, alcohol, sex, people (dysfunctional relationships), and shopping. Social media, hoarding, helping people to the point of pushing aside one's own needs and feelings, and adrenaline (excitement) are other addictions I have witnessed.

Trauma and lack of self-love and self-esteem are often the most important root causes of addictions, partly because they happen long before the addiction begins, and also because they are more difficult to treat than the physical aspects of the addiction. Another root cause of addiction is mental illness, especially depression and anxiety. The powerful emotions in these conditions can be so unpleasant and frightening that a person will do anything to escape them. Focusing obsessively on the object of the addiction is an excellent form of escape, at

least in the beginning. Eventually, the addiction becomes even
more painful and problematic than the feelings the person was
trying to escape from. Of course, addiction doesn't erase the
original feelings, either, so the issues are compounded. Unless
the underlying emotional and spiritual issues are addressed,
permanent healing is nearly impossible.

My recommendation is to find an excellent therapist, one
who is familiar with the spiritual and emotional root causes
of addiction. Jungian counselors are a great fit. It can also be
helpful to use cognitive behavioral therapy and EMDR, or eye
movement desensitization training, for trauma. Twelve-step
programs for addiction, and programs that address dysfunctional family issues are useful for relinquishing control, creating a sense of community and support, and connecting with
Spirit or a higher power. Perfectionism is a key component
of addictive behavior that many people are not aware of. Addicts are incredibly afraid of making mistakes or being seen
as weak, so they often isolate and have significant trust issues.
They see control as a way of not letting anyone else see their
true, flawed self so the concept of a higher power, as used in
twelve-step programs, is essential. Embracing a higher power
is a way to begin trusting a protective, loving force that can
be a source of support and guidance, and can help the addict
feel like they are not alone. ACOA (Adult Children of Alcoholics) is a support group that was very helpful for me, even
though we didn't have alcoholism in my family. Dysfunctional families with all types of addiction issues share similar
characteristics.

Important parts of recovery can include exercise, mindfulness, and other forms of meditation; stress reduction like
massage; a healthy, nontoxic diet with adequate amounts of
complete protein for amino acids that help make neurotransmitters; energy healing, like Reiki; testing for vitamin and
mineral deficiencies; homeopathy; and acupuncture.

ADRENAL GLANDS
Chakras 7, 5, 4, 3

Adrenals are the parts of the body that react when we are faced with danger. They are called the "flight-or-fight" glands. Unfortunately, the majority of people in our fast-paced and stressful world are unable or unwilling to relax. They are dealing with trauma and addiction, often with very little support from others. They do not get enough exercise or other stress relief, and they are exposed to or ingest chemicals, hormones, and other potential toxins. This means that not only are their adrenal glands overstimulated, but that the body systems that support the adrenals are also not functioning at optimum capacity.

Symptoms of adrenal insufficiency include the following:

- Fatigue
- Body aches
- Unexplained weight loss
- Low blood pressure
- Light-headedness
- Loss of body hair
- Skin discoloration (hyperpigmentation)

Adrenal fatigue is not a diagnosis recognized by traditional medicine, but some studies have shown a correlation between the symptoms listed here and subclinical hyper- or hypo-adrenalism (adrenal dysfunction).[9]

To be identified with a recognized adrenal abnormality, blood levels of cortisol must be very low or very high. Many alternative practitioners, along with myself, realize that there is a spectrum of adrenal symptoms. In addition, traditional medicine normally uses a blood test at a single point in time to identify levels of cortisol, thus adrenal function. This test is most accurate if done in the morning, around 8:00 or 8:30, when cortisol is highest, and on an empty stomach. Too many physicians aren't aware of this.

Many alternative practitioners agree that a single blood test does not accurately depict adrenal function and recommend saliva or urine tests done over a twenty-four-hour period. These have been most accurate for me and many of my clients.

Hypoadrenalism is treated with prescription cortisol, but there are many natural ways to support your adrenals and your body's reaction to stress:

- Keep blood sugar steady with small meals including fat and proteins.
- Keep caffeine to a minimum and don't consume it on an empty stomach; including fat and/or protein with caffeine helps to slow absorption (having cream in your coffee is not enough).
- Keep blood pressure steady and avoid blood pressure that is too low or too high.
- Meditate in whatever form that feels good to you; traditional meditation is very effective but so is walking meditation, being in nature, and breathing exercises.
- Exercise, but not excessively. Too much physical movement is taxing on the adrenals. Rest between workouts is important.
- Implement other forms of stress reduction, including creative activities, movement, and dance.
- Perform energy healing exercises.
- Have acupuncture treatment.
- Eliminate chemicals from your diet and environment.
- Eat foods high in vitamin C, B vitamins, and magnesium.
- Stay hydrated.
- Get enough sleep.
- Add supplements to your diet, including licorice root, ash-

wagandha, rhodiola and maca, which are herbs commonly used for stress relief, and Siberian ginseng; also try an adrenal glandular supplement. (Start low and slow with all of these, with the help of a healthcare professional. If you experience symptoms such as fatigue, nervousness, or heart palpitations, reduce the dose or discontinue. It is always best to work with a practitioner when supplementing for adrenal health.)

- Address issues with the thyroid; the thyroid and adrenals support each other.
- Address mental health issues and addiction.

ANXIETY AND DEPRESSION
Chakras 7, 6, 5, 4, 3, 2

I've listed anxiety and depression together because so many symptoms and root causes overlap and because these conditions are often present at the same time. It took many years before I realized that anxiety had been causing a great deal of my depression. The exhaustion of always trying to act and feel normal while struggling with anxiety fed into my depression.

Common symptoms include the following:

- Irritability
- Lack of focus
- Shortness of breath
- Heart palpitations
- Aches and pains
- Gut issues
- Acid reflux
- Brain fog and memory issues
- Insomnia or sleeping too much
- Difficulty listening to intuition

- Self-doubt
- Feeling unsafe
- Loss of faith
- Hair loss
- Weight changes and emotional eating
- Hormone imbalances
- Headaches
- Fatigue

The root causes for anxiety and depression include:

- Medication side effects
- Trauma
- Neurological disorders
- Gut imbalance and not absorbing nutrients correctly (Most of our neurochemicals are made in the gut, not the brain.)
- Poor diet and overconsumption of caffeine
- Other mental health issues
- Addiction
- General stress
- Family history
- Autoimmune condition
- Lyme disease or mold toxicity
- Parasites
- Hormonal imbalance

Psychiatric medications have been the first line of defense in traditional medicine, but these drugs, while they have their place in some cases, are often ineffective and have potentially dangerous and difficult side effects. Medications for anxiety are addictive, and antidepressants, while not technically considered addictive, can be extremely difficult to stop taking and must be slowly tapered off with medical supervision because of serious withdrawal symptoms.

The other important issue with medications is that many people have situational, not biochemical, depression and anxiety. This means that they have valid reasons for their feelings, and these feelings should be addressed, not pushed down with often numbing medication. If people are numb, they cannot attend to the behaviors, situations, and people that are creating emotional pain, and these situations may just get worse.

In addition to seeking therapy, coaching, or getting other psychological support to address issues, these practices can also help:

- Eat a very healthy diet, avoiding sugar, empty calories, alcohol, too much caffeine, and inflammatory foods like gluten and dairy. Food is medicine.

- Exercise. Our feelings are stored in our bodies as energy and this energy needs to be released.

- Remove unhealthy people from your life.

- Practice self-love and self-care.

- Support your adrenal glands. If we are always in fight-or-flight mode, we never give our adrenals a chance to catch up. Supportive herbs include ashwagandha, rhodiola, ginseng, valerian root for relaxation. You may find that a low dose of an over-the-counter adrenal glandular supplement can also be helpful. All of these can be potent, so start low under the supervision of a health professional, and pay attention to any potential side effects. (For more information on supporting adrenal glands, see that entry in this glossary.)

- Remove toxins from your body, food, and environment.

- Be evaluated for possible underlying conditions, such as Lyme disease, mold toxicity, parasites, blood-sugar issues, autoimmune disease, and hormonal imbalances. All of these can cause both anxiety and depression. When the Lyme disease in my body was eradicated, the depression I had suffered with most of my life disappeared, as did most of the anxiety.

- Support gut health with strains of probiotics found to support mental health, like *B. (Bifidobacterium) longum, B. bifidum, B. infantis, and L. (Lactobacillus) reuteri, L. planterum, and L. acidophilus.* Probiotics are naturally found in foods like yogurt and fermented foods also, but I have found that it is especially beneficial to seek out these specific strains. I am very encouraged by studies currently being conducted by prestigious hospitals regarding the use of microdosing mushrooms and other psychedelics. I have clients who live in countries where microdosing is legal. They have successfully used mushrooms for mental illness symptom relief and withdrawal symptoms from antidepressants.

ASTHMA
Chakras 6, 4

Asthma is unfortunately very common, with over 24.5 million people in the United States diagnosed as of 2018 and a U.S. death rate of 10.5 people per million.

Spiritually, the lungs relate to the beginning of life. When babies take their first breath on their own, they are no longer dependent on their mother's body and breath. Asthma relates to not being able to adequately take in the breath of life. It's about feeling trapped, not being able to fully express yourself, and not feeling safe, since we commonly hold our breath when we are afraid or stressed.

Asthma symptoms are often caused by allergies and exposure to allergens, such as pet dander, dust mites, pollen, or mold. Nonallergic triggers include smoke, pollution, cold air, or changes in weather.

Risk factors include the following:

- Exposure to cigarette smoke in the womb or in a child's first few years raises the risk of developing asthma symptoms early in life.
- Exposure to different microbes, including viral bronchitis, strep throat, influenza, mycoplasma pneumonia and chlamydia pneumonia, and rhinoviruses, especially early in life, can increase the risk of developing asthma or exacerbate existing asthma.
- Cesarean deliveries can put children at greater risk because they do not receive the same immune system protections and probiotics as a child delivered vaginally.
- Exposure to chemical irritants or industrial dusts may also raise the risk of developing asthma in susceptible people. This type of asthma is called occupational asthma. It may develop over a period of years, and it often lasts, even once you are no longer exposed.
- Poor air quality from pollution, mold, or allergens may make asthma worse.
- Genetic predisposition can be a factor, especially if the mother has asthma.
- There is an increased risk for asthma due to obesity.
- Among children, more boys have asthma, but among teens and adults it is more common in women.

Possible treatments:[10] There is no cure for asthma, but symptoms can be controlled with effective asthma treatment and management. It involves learning to avoid triggers. You may choose to take inhalers, but most contain corticosteroids, which unfortunately can negatively impact your immune system and your adrenal glands.

Natural treatments include:

- An anti-inflammatory diet that includes plenty of fruits and vegetables, which are great sources of antioxidants and may help reduce inflammation around your airways.
- Other antioxidants including zinc and selenium. High amounts of antioxidants are found in tea (especially green tea), red wine, dark chocolate, coffee, cloves, mint, oregano, garlic, ginger, and allspice. Sangre de grado, an herb made from the sap of a tree found in Peru; the Ayurvedic remedies trehala, arjuna bark extract and Goshuyu-tou, a traditional kampo remedy used in Japanese medicine, are also very high in antioxidants.
- Omega-3 oils, which can be found in fish and flaxseed, have been shown to have many health benefits. They may also work to decrease airway inflammation and improve lung function in people with severe asthma.
- Caffeine, which is a bronchodilator and can reduce respiratory muscle fatigue. Studies have shown that caffeine can be effective for people with asthma. It may be able to improve the function of airways for up to four hours after consumption.[11]
- Osteopathic or chiropractic adjustments, which can properly align the body and perhaps open airways.
- Yoga, which incorporates stretching and breathing exercises to help boost flexibility and increase your overall fitness. For many people, practicing yoga can decrease stress, which may trigger your asthma. The breathing techniques utilized in yoga may also help to reduce the frequency of asthma attacks. However, there isn't currently any conclusive evidence to prove this.
- Hypnotherapy and hypnosis, which are used to make a person more relaxed and open to new ways to think, feel, and behave. Hypnotherapy may help facilitate muscle relaxation,

which may help people with asthma cope with symptoms like chest tightness.[12]

- Mindfulness, which is a type of meditation that focuses on how the mind and the body are feeling in the present moment. It can be practiced almost anywhere. All that you need is a quiet place to sit down, close your eyes, and focus your attention on the thoughts, feelings, and sensations in your body. Because of its stress-relieving benefits, mindfulness can help to complement your prescription medication and relieve stress-related asthma symptoms.

- Acupuncture, a form of ancient Chinese medicine that involves placing small needles into specific points on the body. Long-term benefits of acupuncture have not yet been proven to be effective against asthma. But some people with asthma do find that acupuncture helps to improve airflow and manage symptoms like chest pain.

- Speleotherapy, which involves spending time in a salt room to introduce tiny particles of salt into the respiratory system. Several studies have shown that this can be helpful for the short-term treatment of asthma.[13]

AUTOIMMUNE DISEASE
Chakra 1 and the Chakras of the Specific Body Parts
Impacted by the Autoimmune Condition

Autoimmune disease is basically when the body's immune system becomes overactive and attacks itself. There are more than eighty different types of autoimmune disorders with varying symptoms and severity, even within the same disorder. The exact cause is unknown, but genetic predisposition, inflammation, exposure to toxins, viruses and bacteria, and nutritional deficiency can be contributing factors. The disease my mother contracted from the flu shot, Guillain-Barré syndrome, is an autoimmune disorder, which can be caused by not only vaccines, but also food poisoning and stomach viruses. Many people have more than one autoimmune condition, since having one can put you at additional risk for contracting others.

Having an autoimmune condition doesn't have to negatively impact your quality of life, and many people go through life with very few symptoms, never having been diagnosed. Hashimoto's and Graves' disease are autoimmune disorders that affect the thyroid, often without symptoms or with minimal symptoms in certain people, but with significant symptoms in others. Autoimmune diseases of the skin include potentially less serious disorders like psoriasis, as well as more debilitating issues like vitiligo, alopecia, blistering diseases, and scleroderma. Many people are not aware that type 1 diabetes, certain forms of arthritis, celiac disease, types of anemia, and some cardiac conditions are also autoimmune.

Many people have had success naturally treating autoimmune diseases and their symptoms with anti-inflammatory, autoimmune diets, avoiding toxins, reducing stress and anxiety, healing bacteria and viruses, mindfulness meditation, exercise, and using homeopathic remedies. There are medications for many autoimmune conditions, but they are expensive and can be highly toxic with serious side effects. They only offer quick fixes for the symptoms; they do not address the root causes.

Supplements that can be helpful for symptoms of autoimmune disease are as follows:

- Glutathione—helps with detoxing
- Curcumin—natural anti-inflammatory
- Resveratrol—antioxidant
- Colostrum—made from the milk produced in early breast feeding; strengthens the immune system
- L-glutamine—strengthens the walls of the intestines and stomach; helps with nutrient absorption, irritable bowel syndrome, celiac symptoms

- Vitamin D—strengthens immune response
- Omega-3— helps to lower inflammation; pay attention to the amount of the active ingredients, EPA and DHA, not the number of milligrams of omega-3
- Probiotics—should look for the strains recommended for your particular condition
- L-carnitine—People with celiac are often deficient in this amino acid
- Boswellia—helpful for chronic inflammation
- Peony—paeoniflorin—also helpful for chronic inflammation

Spiritually, autoimmunity can be thought of as a self-attack, often brought on by low self-esteem, negative self-talk or the negative words of others, not feeling like you deserve love or happiness, and self-sabotage. It is not uncommon for me to encounter autoimmune disease in people who have survived but not completely processed trauma, especially abuse, as well as those with addiction including eating disorders, people who engage in self-harm, and those from dysfunctional family backgrounds.

BACKACHE
Chakra 2

Spiritually, the back is about feeling supported, so if you have back issues, consider whether or not you are receiving support from others and if you have in the past. Also think about how you are supporting yourself. I have learned that one of the best things you can do for a strong, pain-free back is to stretch the muscles of your upper and lower back and strengthen your entire body, especially your core, shoulders, and arms. Don't forget your hips and hip flexors. If you are not open and flexible in the hip area, the muscles of the upper and lower back need to compensate, especially while twisting. Many people are not aware of the connection.

This should be done safely and with supervision, like with a trainer or physical therapist, especially if you have back pain, as poor form can cause more problems. Many people injure their backs because they don't have the strength in their arms, shoulders, and core to lift properly or because they twist sideways without having the flexibility to protect the muscles in the back. For treatment and continued back health, I am also a supporter of chiropractic, acupuncture, and energy healing like Reiki.

It is absolutely possible to heal from even the most complicated and painful of back problems. I have the pleasure of knowing an inspirational young woman who has overcome severe back issues. She had scoliosis that required her to have spinal-fusion surgery. In spite of that, she became a gymnast and an accomplished pole athlete, which is how I met her. She began pole as part of the recovery process from one of her surgeries, and now the flexibility in her spine is remarkable.

BLADDER AND CYSTITIS
Chakra 2

The purpose of the bladder is to store and release waste. If you are having issues with this area, think about what "waste" you are carrying and the blocks you have about releasing it. Spiritual waste can include fear, negative messages from yourself and others, and false beliefs.

Cystitis is an inflammation of the bladder, with interstitial cystitis being a chronic inflammation, which is painful, frustrating, and stubborn to treat. Inflammation in this area is most commonly caused by a bacterial imbalance or urinary-tract infection, but it can also be caused by side effects of certain treatments, like radiation, hygiene products like spermicides, feminine hygiene sprays, and exposure to artificial fragrances, like in bubble bath or scented tampons, so it is helpful to eliminate as many chemicals as possible.

When working with people with interstitial cystitis, my guides often bring up hormone imbalances that can cause changes in pH balance and dryness. There is scientific evidence that links birth control to cystitis, and also the hormonal changes that take place during perimenopause and menopause. Testing for hormone levels and treatment with bioidentical hormones that closely mimic those found naturally in the body have been helpful. Cystitis also seems to be linked to high amounts of stress, so meditation and other forms of stress reduction are suggested.

BLOOD DISEASES, ANEMIA, AND LOW FERRITIN
Chakra 1 and Possibly 4

There are many types of blood disorders, some with very serious, debilitating symptoms, and others that many people don't even realize they have that are usually easily treated, such as anemia. They vary greatly in complexity and methods of treatment.

Spiritually, blood is our life force. Red is the color of anger, passion, excitement, and potential danger, for example on a stop sign. Blood diseases may signify a loss of passion and excitement or a belief that life is no longer worth living. They may be warnings to release anger and other emotions and to move forward with life or to stop the way you have been conducting your life and to listen to your intuition and take better care of yourself. High blood pressure can be about "waiting to blow," while low blood pressure can be about feeling emotionally weak or not empowered. Low blood pressure can result in light-headedness and dizziness, which can signal a lack of ability to find focus or direction. Anemia can be a sign that you feel weak or powerless, while low ferritin can be spiritually related to not recognizing your own power or not having it recognized by others for an extended length of time.

When addressing blood diseases, pay attention to the individual symptoms and organs that are affected. They often apply to more than one chakra.

Anemia occurs when you do not have enough healthy red blood cells to bring adequate oxygen to your body's organs and tissues. Ferritin is a blood protein that contains iron, and ferritin levels refer to iron storage. It is possible to not have anemia but to have low ferritin. Low ferritin and anemia are common conditions that many people are not even aware they have. They can cause fatigue, impaired thyroid function, irritability, anxiety, depression, leg pain, dizziness, low blood pressure, lack of stamina, decreased hair growth or hair loss, headaches, and ringing in the ears, among other symptoms.

Most medical professionals don't even test for ferritin, especially traditional medical professionals. I have almost always had to ask for it. One of the problems with testing is that the "normal" range is from 12 to 150 ng (nanograms) per ml (milliliter) for women and 12 to 300 mg per ml for men. I have been advised by numerous medical practitioners, and it has been my experience that the optimal ferritin levels are between 50 and 70 ng per ml for both men and women. This is supported in a May 2019 article in the *Journal of the American Academy of Dermatology* as well.

It can be difficult to obtain adequate iron from food, especially if you are vegetarian or vegan, since iron from animal sources is 33 percent more absorbable. Certain vegetables that are high in iron, like spinach, contain other compounds, called polyphenols, that inhibit iron absorption. Only 1.7 percent of the iron in spinach is actually absorbed, as compared to 20 percent of the iron in sirloin steak.[14] If you need supplementation, which many people, including vegans, do, the best sources are from heme iron, which is derived from animal sources, but ferrous bisglycinate is also highly absorbable and not made from animals. Look for supplements that also include vitamin C, which helps with absorption.

Supplementation with iron can be problematic since it can sometimes cause constipation. You never want to supplement unless you have tested to confirm low iron or ferritin, and you should retest on a regular basis. High ferritin can cause organ damage, stomach pain, heart palpitations, weakness and fatigue, and joint pain.

BONES
Chakra 1

Think that bone density is something only older people need to be concerned with? Bone loss typically begins at age thirty and is impacted by what you do at every age, even your teens and twenties.[15] Osteoporosis (brittle bones and bone loss) is defined as having a "T score" of –2.5. A T score is a number comparing bone density to people of the same age with healthy bones. Osteopenia, a precursor, has a T score of –1 to –2.4. Often, people are not even aware that they have low bone density until they have a bone fracture, lose height, or develop curvature of the spine.

Prevention and early detection are important, especially since bone density medication can cause serious side effects. According to the National Osteoporosis Foundation, these symptoms include muscle pain, nausea, flulike symptoms, difficulty swallowing, gastric ulcers, inflammation of the eye, kidney function changes, and bone fracture.[16]

Women are more likely to experience bone density issues than men because they tend to have lighter and smaller bones. According to the National Institute of Health, conditions that increase a person's risk for low bone density include the following:

- Eating disorders
- Heavy alcohol use

- Celiac disease
- Radiation treatment
- Family history of osteoporosis
- Poor nutrition
- Smoking
- Lack of exercise
- Low estrogen and testosterone
- Certain autoimmune conditions
- Thyroid medications
- Corticosteroids
- PCOS (polycystic ovary syndrome)

What can be done to prevent and treat low bone density naturally?

- Quit or at least reduce smoking.
- Reduce alcohol consumption.
- Do weight bearing exercises and lift weights. Not only does this help your bones and muscles, it helps you feel strong and empowered. After a year of taking pole dancing and stretch classes several times a week, my bone density went from a T score of –1.2 to –0.8.
- Get scanned for bone density. It is typically recommended beginning at age fifty or after menopause or earlier if you have had your ovaries surgically removed. If you are taking thyroid medication or have any of the risk factors listed, you may want to request bone density scanning earlier than age fifty.
- Discuss hormone replacement if you are peri- or post-menopausal. Many practitioners can treat with bioidentical hormones, rather than synthetic. Women who are estrogen-receptive are usually advised not to use hormone replacement therapy and should consult their physician before doing so.

- Eat a diet high in calcium, vitamin D, magnesium, DHA (found in fish oil), and vitamin K. Sunshine is an excellent source of vitamin D as well, and you only need ten to thirty minutes of midday sun, several times a week. You can also try strontium ranelate, a mineral that has been found to be effective for preventing and treating bone loss. Strontium ranelate has been approved for this purpose in the United Kingdom but not in the United States, and there is controversy about its effectiveness and potentially serious side effects.

- Pay attention to gut health. A healthy gut allows you to absorb vitamins and minerals properly.

- Avoid the use of steroids, especially long term. These are commonly found in nasal sprays, even over-the-counter products. Investigate natural, effective ways of treating and preventing allergy and sinus symptoms.

- Inquire about bone density issues in your family

It is possible to treat and prevent bone loss naturally and it is never too early to start.

Spiritually, strong bones are about having a strong support system and having "a backbone." People with bone density issues or curvature of the spine may not feel supported by family and friends. They may have trouble "standing up for themselves" and being seen.

BREAST CANCER
Chakras 7, 4

A spiritual trait I encounter frequently in people who have had breast cancer is the intense need to take care of others and to relieve their pain, often to the detriment of themselves. It can be very difficult for these people to watch others suffering because they feel it so deeply themselves and haven't been taught how to establish boundaries. They may have learned this in dysfunctional family situations involving addiction, narcissism, or mental illness of parents who expected everyone else to serve them and anticipate their every need. If the other members of the household didn't comply, they would face anger, rejection, ridicule, and even abuse.

When you grow up like this, you aren't encouraged or even allowed to have opinions, needs, or wants. You certainly aren't taught how to listen to intuition or trust yourself. It is exactly the opposite. You learn that your identity, and the way you achieve the love of others, is to put your own needs aside and take care of everyone else. Healing from breast cancer, and many other diseases, means putting your old, outdated beliefs aside and changing how you think about and interact with the world.

PTSD often comes along with breast or any other type of cancer. This can be a result of difficult and often painful treatments and surgeries, but I find most often that it is because of a fear that the cancer will return. Traditional medicine tells cancer patients that their cancer is "in remission," which seems to imply that it is just a matter of time before it comes back. Patients fear that if they don't constantly worry about it and watch for signs, they will go through the same trauma all over again.

It is known that stress contributes to inflammation, damages the immune system, and is linked to cancer. It is linked to emotional eating as well, which often consists of eating unhealthy, sugary foods. Stress is the opposite of what people who have survived cancer need.

I encourage people who have survived cancer or any type of illness that "might return" to think of themselves as healed and healthy. Letting go of expectations and fears of certain doom means that they can think about today, not the past or the future. They can and should still get scanned or checked, but they cannot be ruled by fear.

I believe that the decisions about treatment need to be made by the person who has the disease and their families. Fortunately, more and more cancer hospitals are offering holistic care along with traditional treatments, which I think is very important.

CARDIOVASCULAR DISEASE
Chakra 4 and Possibly 1 If the Disease Is Autoimmune

Statistically, men are more likely to die from a cardiovascular event than women are, and cardiovascular disease develops seven to ten years earlier in men than in women.[17] These statistics have been narrowing, but I believe that the discrepancy is because, traditionally, men have not been encouraged to share their feelings or to be sensitive. As I have said, emotions not expressed in a healthy manner become buried and are then expressed by the body in unhealthy ways.

Many cardiovascular conditions are autoimmune, including: rheumatic fever; pericarditis, or inflammation in the sac surrounding the heart; myocarditis, which is inflammation in the heart muscle; endocarditis, or inflammation in the hearts' inner walls and valves; and coronary artery disease, narrowed blood vessels due to fatty deposits.

In addition, many autoimmune diseases such as lupus, scleroderma, and psoriasis may have cardiac-related symptoms and may increase the risk of cardiac disease.

It is widely known that exercise, stress relief including meditation, a healthy diet, reducing cholesterol, quitting smoking, and reducing alcohol consumption help lower the risk of heart disease and can prevent it from worsening.

Many natural remedies have been found to be helpful with cardiovascular disease, but consult with your health-care practitioner before trying them, because some, like garlic, may interact with medications like blood thinners. Remedies include the following:

- Coenzyme Q-10 (CoQ10)
- Red yeast rice
- Flaxseed
- Vitamin K2
- Resveratrol and other polyphenols
- Herbs used in Chinese medicine, including hawthorn and motherwort
- Acupuncture

Spiritually, the heart is the seat of affections. It is where we process emotion, especially love and hate. There are recognized cases of partners passing away of broken hearts shortly after the other has died. Self-love is an important part of physical heart health and of healthy circulation, because a lack of love has the potential to energetically block any of the chakras, thus blocking the flow of life force, or chi.

CHRONIC FATIGUE SYNDROME
Chakras 7, 3, 1

There are so many causes for fatigue, and the most important way to start treating it is to determine the root cause or causes. Possible causes include the following:

- Food intolerances.
- Nutritional components of food consumed: Too many carbohydrates and too little protein and fat are common culprits. I usually advise that people consume some protein and/or fat when they eat carbs, because these combinations help

to keep blood sugar (and energy) even by preventing the crash that often happens after carbohydrate intake.

- Dehydration: Many people are dehydrated and do not realize it.

- Caffeine: While it is true that caffeine temporarily increases energy, we often crash a few hours later, setting up the need for more caffeine. It can also interfere with sleep and create dehydration because it is a diuretic. Eating protein and/or fat with caffeine can help slow or prevent this crash.

- Overworked or inactive adrenals: please see the section on adrenal glands in this glossary.

- Depression and anxiety: Aside from the fact that fatigue is a symptom of both of these issues, it is also exhausting to constantly try to feel good and present a "happy face."

- Sleep issues: This is a no brainer, however many people think that they are sleeping well but actually are not. Go to bed by 10 P.M. each night and wake up at a regular time each day. Pay attention to your individual need for sleep. My husband only needs five or six hours (so jealous), while I need at least eight.

- Stress: Without stress reduction, the worries and pressures of the day build up in our bodies and physically, emotionally, and spiritually wear us out.

- Lack of exercise: While fatigue may reduce your motivation and energy to move, without movement our metabolisms plummet and we feel tired.

- Nutrient absorption or lack of nutrition: We need a bare minimum of the RDA (recommended dietary allowance) of vitamins and minerals as well as complete proteins with amino acids. Our bodies cannot make most of these on their own. There are various reasons why people cannot absorb or process nutrients, like genetic conditions, such as MTHFR, or gut issues. MTHFR stands for methylene tetrahydrofolate reductase and mutations in these genes can alter the processing of folate and other nutrients and can make normal detoxing more difficult.

- Underactive thyroid or autoimmune thyroid conditions: these could possibly be caused by low iodine.
- Hormone imbalances: These can happen at any age, not just before or after menopause.
- Underlying viruses like those responsible for chronic fatigue virus and Epstein-Barr.
- Various autoimmune conditions.
- Side effects of medications or supplements.
- Lack of creative expression.
- Boredom and not being fulfilled.

Spiritually, chronic fatigue is a way of shutting down and tuning out. It makes you more present and mindful, because you can't continue to live at the rapid pace you may have sustained before the fatigue set in. When you are continually on the go, it is very difficult to connect to your body, your intuition, or psychic abilities; so if you are dealing with chronic fatigue, ask yourself if you need to pay more attention to your health and to your spiritual life. Ask yourself if there is anything you have been afraid to face or have been "running away from," such as unhappy relationships or an unfulfilling job.

COLD FEET AND/OR HANDS
Chakra 1

Cold feet and hands can be indicative of an autoimmune condition impacting circulation, called Raynaud's disease. There is no known cure, but anything that improves circulation, like exercise and deep breathing, can help. The origin is also not known, but this disease primarily impacts girls and women and can happen after an injury, as a result of smoking, or exposure to certain drugs and toxic chemicals. A great source of additional information is at www.Raynauds.org.[18]

Spiritually, cold feet or hands can mean exactly that: fear, resistance, and holding back.

DIABETES, HYPOGLYCEMIA, AND INSULIN RESISTANCE
Chakras 7, 3, 1

Diabetes is an elevation of blood sugar, and hypoglycemia is a reduction in blood sugar, both at abnormal levels. Hypoglycemia may also be referred to as an insulin reaction or insulin shock. It can happen in conjunction with or separately from diabetes.

Insulin resistance is a condition in which the body's cells don't respond normally to insulin, and this can be a precursor to getting diabetes. Diabetes is common; the CDC estimates that in 2018, 34.5 percent of people in the United States (over 10 percent of the population) had this condition. There are over three million cases of insulin resistance diagnosed in the United States per year.

Blood sugar in the body is controlled by the pancreas. The spiritual symbolism of the pancreas has to do with the sweetness of life, how much you are enjoying or not happy with your life, along with resentments and taking responsibility for your life circumstances. It's important to feel empowered and to have a positive outlook in general, and this will especially benefit the health of your pancreas.

Diabetes is an autoimmune disease, which many people are not aware of. It occurs when the immune system attacks the insulin producing cells in the pancreas. Spiritually, autoimmune diseases are about self-attack, since autoimmune literally means "the immune system attacking itself" (read more about autoimmune disease under that entry in this glossary).

Diabetes is also related to the liver because that is where glucose is processed. In traditional Chinese medicine, the liver is connected to anger and the flow of emotions. If you are holding on to anger, toward others or yourself, you are more likely to have a liver that doesn't function efficiently.

There are two types of diabetes, type 1 and type 2. People with type 1 do not make insulin, and those with type 2 do not process insulin correctly and may eventually not be able to make it at all as the disease progresses. According to research and traditional medical beliefs, type 1 isn't preventable, while type 2 is. The cause of type 1 diabetes isn't known, but it is thought to be a combination of genetic predisposition and environmental factors.

There are many diseases, including many mental health conditions, whose causes are also unknown but are thought to be a combination of genetic predisposition and environmental factors. We know that children who grow up in stressful, economically deprived, environmentally toxic, and trauma-filled homes are more likely to develop depression, anxiety, ADHD, and other issues, while the opposite is true for children who grow up in more stable and healthy households. While diabetes is certainly a different condition from these mental health issues, I believe that diabetes and other autoimmune conditions would be much less likely to develop in children raised under healthy, nurturing circumstances.

From milder, more common indicators to most severe signs, symptoms of low blood sugar include the following:[19]

- Feeling shaky
- Being nervous or anxious
- Sweating, chills, and clamminess
- Irritability or impatience

- Confusion
- Increase in heartrate
- Feeling light-headed or dizzy
- Hunger
- Nausea
- Color draining from the skin (pallor)
- Feeling sleepy
- Feeling weak or having no energy
- Blurred/impaired vision
- Tingling or numbness in the lips, tongue, or cheeks
- Headaches
- Coordination problems, clumsiness
- Nightmares or crying out during sleep
- Seizures

The only sure way to know whether you are experiencing low blood sugar is to check your blood sugar, if possible. If you are experiencing symptoms and you are unable to check your blood sugar for any reason, treat the hypoglycemia. Most people with this condition are well aware of its onset before they ever check their blood-sugar levels.

A low blood-sugar level triggers the release of epinephrine (adrenaline), the fight-or-flight hormone. Epinephrine is what can cause the symptoms of hypoglycemia, such as increased heartbeat, sweating, tingling, and anxiety.

If the blood-sugar level continues to drop, the brain does not get enough glucose and stops functioning as it should. This can lead to blurred vision, difficulty concentrating, confused thinking, slurred speech, numbness, and drowsiness. If blood sugar stays low for too long, starving the brain of glucose, it may lead to seizures, coma, and very rarely death.

Risk factors for developing type 1 diabetes include:

- Family history
- Environmental factors like exposure to certain viruses, including enteroviruses, such as Coxsackievirus B (CVB), but also rotavirus, mumps virus, and cytomegalovirus, both in utero and as children[20]
- The presence of diabetes autoantibodies

Risk factors for type 2 diabetes, insulin resistance, and hypoglycemia include:

- Weight: The more fatty tissue you have, the more resistant your cells become to insulin.
- Inactivity: The less active you are, the greater your risk. Physical activity helps you control your weight, uses up glucose as energy, and makes your cells more sensitive to insulin.
- Family history: Your risk increases if a parent or sibling has type 2 diabetes.
- Race: Although it's unclear why, people of certain races—including black people, Hispanics, American Indians, and Asian Americans—are at higher risk.
- Age: Your risk increases as you get older. This may be because you tend to exercise less, lose muscle mass, and gain weight as you age. But type 2 diabetes is also increasing among children, adolescents, and younger adults.
- Gestational diabetes: If you developed gestational diabetes when you were pregnant, your risk of developing prediabetes and type 2 diabetes later increases. If you gave birth to a baby weighing more than nine pounds (four kilograms), you're also at risk of type 2 diabetes.
- Polycystic ovary syndrome: For women, having polycystic ovary syndrome—a common condition characterized by irregular menstrual periods, excess hair growth, and obesity—increases the risk of diabetes.

- High blood pressure: Having blood pressure over 140/90 millimeters of mercury (mm Hg) is linked to an increased risk of type 2 diabetes.

- Abnormal cholesterol and triglyceride levels: If you have low levels of high-density lipoprotein (HDL), or "good" cholesterol, your risk of type 2 diabetes is higher. Triglycerides are another type of fat carried in the blood. People with high levels of triglycerides have an increased risk of type 2 diabetes. Your doctor can order a blood test and let you know what your cholesterol and triglyceride levels are.

It makes sense that treatment of these risk factors helps to both treat blood-sugar abnormalities as well as prevent them.[21] Many patients turn to medications, but those can have serious side effects.

Natural ways to fight diabetes, insulin resistance, and hypoglycemia include:

- Adequate sleep
- Avoiding stress
- Exercise
- Eating a low-carbohydrate diet, along with eating protein and/or fat when you eat carbohydrates or caffeine (this helps to maintain even blood sugar, avoiding the rapid rise after carbohydrate and caffeine consumption, followed by a crash)
- Maintaining a healthy weight
- Getting adequate fiber in the diet
- Using the herbs fenugreek, turmeric, ginger, garlic, and cinnamon
- Studies have shown that green tea, apple cider vinegar, and the supplements chromium, magnesium, resveratrol, and berberine are also helpful. It is always best to get your nutrients from

food, but if you use supplements, it is helpful to do so under the supervision of a medical professional.

DIET
Chakras 7, 6, 3

I do not recommend one type of diet because I think that we all function differently and need to choose what is appropriate for our bodies. Listen to your body and intuition, and they will tell you what foods are a good fit and which aren't, as well as when you are full, hungry, or thirsty. Most people make it far too complicated and overthink, which creates an atmosphere of anxiety, confusion, and even guilt around eating. There are no good or bad foods. If you crave something, there is a reason. You may be in need of certain nutrients or need foods that help regulate your hormones. You may need to focus or relax, so think about how the food or foods you are wanting may impact your neurochemicals. We make neurochemicals from amino acids, which are found in protein. Not all protein is nutritionally equivalent, though. Complete proteins found in meat, soy, quinoa, buckwheat, hemp, and eggs give us all nine of the amino acids we require that we cannot make on our own. Amino acids create neurochemicals involved in mood, the ability to pay attention, sleep, and more. Carbohydrates and certain other foods, like turkey, which contains tryptophan, help the body produce the neurochemical serotonin, which brings on a relaxation response. If you crave carbohydrates, you may need to support your blood sugar, adrenals, and energy levels. Food is truly medicine.

In general, I find that most people benefit from a primarily plant-based diet with complete proteins, including humanely raised animal proteins, healthy fats, and organically raised grains. If you have any autoimmune conditions, inflammatory conditions, or emotional illness, then a grain-free, non-GMO, and mostly soy-free diet might be more appropriate, but be aware of individual sensitivities, like histamines, yeast, and dairy. Pay attention to how your body responds to dairy products. Many people do not digest it well, especially as we age and produce fewer digestive enzymes. Some people can tolerate goat products or lactose-free products from cattle raised organically, and cows that are not injected with growth hormones, including rBGH (recombinant bovine growth hormone). This hormone has been linked to several forms of cancer and other health risks, according to studies done by Harvard. Since sugar is a natural inflammatory and can impact the quality of our skin and how it ages, aside from being a source of empty calories, I recommend limiting it. As I have said I am a strong advocate of non-toxic living and optimal nutrition, so it's a great idea to eat food that is as fresh and organic as possible. If you choose to be vegan, especially if you are active or if you are trying to lose weight, be sure to get a minimum of the recommended daily amount of *complete* proteins. Most people need more than that to feel energized and to build muscle.

It is important to eat intuitively, since being on a diet often cuts us off from our bodies. We might override hunger, thirst, cravings, and the symptoms that might be created by foods that do not fit our nutritional needs.

EXERCISE AND MOVEMENT
Chakras 7, 6, 4, 3

The key to consistent exercise and movement is to find something you really enjoy so that it doesn't feel like work or "punishment" for being overweight. If your motivation is positive—having more energy, stress relief, building skills, being out in nature, and spending more time with friends or family—you are much more likely to continue and be successful than if you are exercising because you feel like you have to or because you are ashamed of your body.

I started pole dance fitness at the age of fifty-three and I'm now obsessed. I don't think of it as exercise, but I'm more fit and stronger than I have ever been. It was sometimes difficult to motivate myself to go to the gym, and it was usually because I was trying to lose weight or trying to prevent weight gain.

When my daughter started pole dance, I thought it might be fun, because it reminded me of doing gymnastics, which I loved when I was younger. The benefits of pole dancing extend far beyond physical strength. It has improved my memory and mental dexterity, since I have to coordinate the left and right sides of my body, including while hanging upside down, and have to put together a series of movements. I never would have dreamed that I would post public videos of myself in basically a bikini, especially at a higher weight than I have been in a very long time, and actually liking the way my stronger, more muscular body looks.

I cannot recommend exercise and movement enough for stress relief, improved bone and immune health, a stronger heart, better circulation and digestion, more restful sleep, and mental clarity. Physical strength helps to build emotional strength and a sense of security and confidence. It becomes a form of meditation, as you must focus on what you are doing now, rather than be preoccupied with thoughts of the past or future you can't control. Exercise can also be a great way to build community, whether that be friends at a yoga studio or a running club. It doesn't matter what you do, just move.

FERTILITY AND SEXUAL DYSFUNCTION
Chakra 2

Often, when people come to me with fertility or sexual dysfunction issues, it is because traditional medical interventions have not been successful. I explore nutritional absorption and related root causes, the possibility of fibroids or endometriosis (which can be difficult to detect and treat), a history of eating disorders or excessive dieting, hormone imbalances, genetic factors, and trauma, especially related to sexual abuse and assault.

It's also important to consider emotional and spiritual root causes. It is not uncommon for me to pick up issues with relationships, careers, and dysfunctional family backgrounds. If you are fearful about the future of your relationship, intuitively know that you need to leave the relationship but have not done so, fear that children will squelch career aspirations, or are afraid of being a "bad" parent because of your own childhood experiences, you may unconsciously be blocking your ability to have children. If you are afraid of being vulnerable and getting close to someone because you have been hurt in the past, being intimate might create intense stress. A natural result of that might be an inability to orgasm or perform sexually.

There are therapists who specialize in issues such as these as well as intimacy. Individual as well as couples therapy could be very beneficial. I recommend doing some of the exercises in previous chapters to connect with your body and improve body image and acceptance. Therapeutic techniques for releasing trauma, such as EMDR, can be helpful as well as physical and emotional stress relief like meditation, movement, and creative activities.

Creativity is a key component of 2nd chakra health, since the uterus is literally where human creation begins. Many people have a fear of creativity because of performance anxiety or a focus on the outcome rather than enjoying the process. We expose vulnerable parts of our inner selves when we produce art, music, engage in dance, and write. This fear can create energy blocks in the 2nd chakra, also potentially blocking fertility.

As we know, our thoughts and feelings are manifested physically if not dealt with emotionally. In addition, stress has been linked to fertility and sexual dysfunction issues in

animals and humans. The anxiety connected with these issues is very stressful.[22]

FIBROMYALGIA
Chakras 7, 6, 1

According to the NIH, symptoms of fibromyalgia are pain and
tenderness throughout your body. Other symptoms may also
include trouble sleeping, morning stiffness, headaches, painful
menstrual periods, tingling or numbness in hands and feet,
and problems with thinking and memory. There are many
people, including myself, who believe that the disease labeled
"fibromyalgia" is actually a symptom of Lyme disease. The
symptoms for fibromyalgia are also symptoms for Lyme.

There are no definitive tests for fibromyalgia, and many
people I have encountered who are diagnosed with it were
given that label because their doctors weren't able to diagnose
them with anything else. Many had Lyme disease tests, which
were negative, but Lyme testing is horribly inaccurate, especially the preliminary tests approved by the CDC, which rec-
ommends more in-depth testing only after the Western blot
test has come back negative. It makes me very upset that so
many people have to suffer for years because of inadequate
testing and uninformed practitioners.

Another issue with fibromyalgia, like other autoimmune
conditions, is that it is strongly linked to Epstein-Barr virus
(EBV) or chronic fatigue syndrome, since the presence of
these can make you more susceptible and make healing more
difficult. If you have received this diagnosis, I recommend that
you see a practitioner who is familiar with all of these conditions, including Lyme disease, to look for underlying root
causes. I also recommend following the recommendations for
autoimmune disease earlier in this glossary.

FOOD ALLERGIES AND INTOLERANCES
Chakras 7, 3, and Those of Any Area of the Body Impacted by the Condition

Every three minutes in the United States, someone goes to the emergency room because of a food allergy reaction with approximately 150–200 deaths each year. Over 170 foods are potential allergens. Food allergies in children have been increasing. The U.S. Centers for Disease Control and Prevention report that food allergies in children in the United States have increased approximately 50 percent between 1997 and 2011, impacting 1 in 13 children. Between 1997 and 2008, the number of nut-related allergies nearly tripled. Adult onset food allergies are also on the rise.[23, 24]

Theories for the reasons why food allergies (and autoimmune conditions) have increased include the "hygiene hypothesis," which refers to a reduced lack of exposure to illness and infectious agents in childhood as well as an increased exposure to antibiotics that kill off the helpful bacteria in our gut. Both of these can cause our immune systems to be either over-reactive or under-reactive. Childhood illness serves the purpose of naturally boosting the immune system, since we are born without them. Vaginal birth and breast feeding help to begin building infant immune systems, but many children are born via cesarean delivery and not all women are able to breast feed. The FDA is investigating this theory. Excessive cleanliness, which lowers the body's exposure to bacteria and viruses and climate change, creating conditions in which plants have longer growing seasons and produce more pollen are also possible reasons for the increase.[25]

Allergies are basically intensified immune reactions and the potential symptoms created by food allergies and intolerances are vast and varied. Aside from rashes, heart palpitations, abdominal pain, changes in bowel movements, and itching, they include the following:

- Headaches
- General aches and pains
- Fatigue
- Heartburn
- Bloating
- Sinus issues
- Symptoms that mimic autoimmune conditions

Food allergies and intolerances can be difficult to diagnose. There are blood tests for things like celiac disease—an allergy to gluten, which test for specific IgEs (Immunoglobulin E antibodies)—and skin testing can help diagnose allergies to many foods and other substances, but intolerances are more difficult. There are various antibody tests available that can be done at home or through alternative practitioners, but they can be expensive and they usually only detect IgG antibodies (Immunoglobulin G) for the top 85 percent of your offenders. They are controversial since there is a lack of reliable evidence about their accuracy. I find that the most accurate way of determining the healthiest foods for you and those that may cause you problems is to eat intuitively.

Before you eat something, hold it in your hand. Ask yourself if it will taste and feel good. If the answer is yes, put it in your mouth and chew it slowly, actively tasting every bite. If it doesn't taste or feel good, do not eat it.

If you do eat the food in question, check in with your body during the process and immediately following, as well as an hour and several hours after. Notice if your mood changes, if you feel tired or energized, if you have a headache or become congested, how your digestive system and throat feel, or if you have any other effects. Write down what happened and keep a journal. Notice what happens the next time you eat the same food and see if a pattern develops. Also make note of the quantity of food you're consuming. I can eat a little dairy without much of an effect, but I am a mess if I eat too much. I can usually tolerate dairy without lactose much better than dairy with lactose.

Also notice what happens if you avoid the offending foods for a while. You may be able to tolerate a particular food occasionally, like once a month, but more than that and it becomes a problem.

Spiritually, allergies are about creating boundaries, or distance, between yourself and the rest of the world. The stronger your boundaries, the less you need to have allergies or sensitivities, because you are already protected. Allergies and sensitivities can warn us about foods and other substances that may do serious harm. If you are reacting to something, think about people or situations that may also be toxic or harmful, especially those that you may have difficulty separating from emotionally or physically.

GALLBLADDER
Chakra 3

The gallbladder's primary function is to store bile, which breaks up fats from the foods we eat. It also drains waste products from the liver into the small intestine. The most common problem with the gallbladder is the formation of stones, which can be painful if they reach a certain size. Surgery may be necessary to remove the gallbladder or the stones, which are created by an excess of cholesterol, bilirubin, or bile salts. Without a gallbladder, it can be difficult to properly digest fats.

So-called gallbladder cleanses likely do not do very much to remove stones and may create unpleasant digestive or bowel symptoms. The gallbladder does benefit from a diet high in fiber, eating healthy fats like olive and avocado oils, and avoiding foods high in unhealthy saturated and trans fats, fats found in meat, full-fat dairy, and hydrogenated fats, as well as maintaining a healthy weight and exercise. I am a huge proponent of acupuncture for the health of organs like the gallbladder and liver as well.

In traditional Chinese medicine, the gallbladder is considered a "curious organ" because it is a yang organ that does not transport impure substances. Yin and yang are concepts in Chinese medicine that describe the notion that everything in nature consists of two inverse phases or energies, with yang meaning masculine, light, activity, and the left side, and yin meaning female, darkness, rest, and the right side. The gallbladder is seen as the turning point for new beginnings and new stages of life. It is responsible for decision-making, judgment, and courage, and when the organ is deficient, fear, lack of initiative, and lack of assertiveness are seen.

Spiritually, this means that when you are having issues with your gallbladder, you should pay attention to new opportunities, relationships, and phases in your life. Be open to them and do not allow fear to prevent you from embracing them. Let your intuition guide you in terms of what you need to release and what toxic emotions or people you might be clinging to.

HEADACHES
Chakras 7, 6, and Whatever Condition the Root Cause of the Headaches Is Related To

The list of possible causes for headaches is extensive and includes the following:

- Autoimmune diseases such as Sjögren's
- Thyroid issues
- Side effects from medication or supplements
- Food intolerances

- Mold
- Sinus problems and allergies
- Magnesium deficiency
- Eyesight issues
- Chemical or toxin exposure
- Hormonal imbalances, sometimes related to the menstrual cycle
- Neurochemical imbalance
- Lyme and related diseases
- Stress and anxiety
- Signal from your intuition (third eye) to pay attention
- Tooth pain, teeth grinding, and jaw alignment issues
- Neck issues
- Concussion
- Brain issues
- Not enough sleep
- Dehydration

It is essential to identify the root causes of headaches and treat these, not just band-aid them with symptom relief. Chiropractors, acupuncturists, and Chinese medicine practitioners can be quite helpful for headaches, including for migraines. Meditation and stress relief are essential, and Botox may also be an option. The headache is most often just a symptom of the underlying cause, which must be treated in order for the headache to subside.

Spiritually I am told by my guides that headaches are a symbol of fighting with ourselves and overthinking. I visualize two boxers fighting to the death, afraid to listen to the ideas of the other because they are ashamed of possibly being wrong. It's related to an inability to trust Spirit and feel safe, and the mistaken assumption that we always need to be in control or our world will fall apart.

Migraines are especially spiritually fascinating because they can cause us to see auras, flashing lights, have distorted vision, cause light-headedness, and immediately force us to stop doing what we were doing because the pain is so intense. They are impossible to ignore, and you instantly have to make yourself a priority and take care of yourself. They remove you from what is happening in your life, which is significant if you are not able to do that for yourself, for instance, if you are feeling helpless to get out of an unhappy relationship or job or if you always put other people before yourself. It is important to pay attention to what is happening in your life when migraines occur, because those events may be physical, emotional, and spiritual triggers. Also consider what is going on when the migraine begins to subside.

Spiritually, think about what the pain might be distracting you from. If the pain is primarily in the front (third-eye area), it could be a signal from your intuition that it would be helpful to connect more to your intuitive abilities and trust the universe. Headaches are often helpful symptoms to alert us to issues and conditions that were present before the headaches started, which can cause serious harm or even death. Many people whom I have worked with never would have discovered brain tumors, autoimmune conditions, seizure disorders, neck and spine issues, and more if it were not because they sought help for the pain in their heads.

HEMORRHOIDS
Chakra 1

Hemorrhoids are not usually serious, and over-the-counter products, increasing the fiber in your diet as well as addressing constipation are often most helpful. Spiritually, a hemorrhoid is a pain in the ass, so think about who or what this might apply to in your life.

HERXING
Could Relate to Any of the Chakras, Depending on the Issue and Parts of the Body Impacted

Negative side effects as a result of toxicity are often mistaken for "herxing," a nickname for a Jarisch-Herxheimer reaction, in which the body becomes overwhelmed by the effects of dying microbes, supposedly a sign that the treatment is working.

There are conditions that can interfere with the body's normal ability to detoxify itself like genetic mutations, liver damage, substance abuse, viruses, exposure to chemicals, and being malnourished. Many people assume that herxing is a necessary part of treatment for Lyme disease and other conditions, but this isn't true. If you are having painful or unpleasant side effects, you should always report these to your practitioner so adjustments can be made to the dosage and intensity of what you are receiving. If you are treating yourself and having negative reactions, it is best to stop and consult with a professional.

HORMONE IMBALANCES
Chakras 7, 6, 3, 2

Hormone imbalance can happen at any age, not just when a woman is close to menopause, and it can cause serious physical, emotional, and even spiritual symptoms, which are often misdiagnosed. The list of symptoms is very long, with some common ones being gut issues like indigestion, constipation, and diarrhea, changes in blood sugar, depression and anxiety, decreased bone density, weight and appetite changes, changes in frequency of urination, headaches, infertility, acne, pain during sex, and bladder infections.

Causes include pregnancy (even years after giving birth), polycystic ovary syndrome; eating disorders; nutritional deficiencies; excessive exercise; supplements, including biotin and saw palmetto, which are taken for hair, skin and nails; soy and other phytoestrogens; chemicals, fragrances, and plastics, which are endocrine disruptors; hormones added to food; perimenopause and menopause; stress; and medications.

It is important to receive a correct diagnosis. Many people are put on psychiatric medications for symptoms that are caused by hormone imbalance. This happened to me. A year and a half after the birth of my older daughter, I started having severe panic attacks, which I later realized was due to postpartum depression. Doctors wanted to put me on psychiatric medications with serious side effects, but low-dose estrogen solved the problem. Blood tests are a start, but they don't tell the whole story, since "normal" isn't the same as optimal. My objective when assisting clients is always improvement in quality of life and how a person feels rather than values on a piece of paper. More in-depth testing, like a DUTCH (dried urine testing for comprehensive hormones) test, can tell you how the hormones are interacting with each other and being processed by the body, so such tests might be more useful. Most traditional medicine doctors don't know what these are.

Spiritually, hormone issues are more about the effects of the imbalance than the hormones themselves. Someone with polycystic ovary syndrome, who produces too much testosterone, could be turning away from the traditionally female aspects of herself, like caretaking, for example. If the imbalance affects fertility, the person could be fearful of being a parent or of responsibility.

Hormones are a complicated topic, so this was a quick overview.

HYPERTENSION AND LOW BLOOD PRESSURE
Chakras 6, 4, 1

Hypertension, or high blood pressure, is commonly and unfortunately most often treated with medications, including diuretics, beta-blockers, antihypertensive drugs, calcium channel blockers, and vasodilators. Side effects from these drugs include fatigue, gout, loss of potassium, impotence, blood-sugar changes, insomnia, depression, kidney damage, loss of taste, headache, constipation, and fluid retention. Much safer and often equally effective treatments are meditation and mindfulness, exercise and other stress reduction, maintaining a healthy weight, a diet low in sodium, avoiding alcohol and inflammatory foods, and quitting smoking.

Spiritually, you can think of high blood pressure as someone getting ready to blow. If you hold in anger, fear, and resentment, or any other feeling, the energy created by these feelings has no outlet and builds up. Because it impacts the heart, hypertension is also related to the 4th chakra so calls to action in that chapter would also be beneficial.

Low blood pressure is often related to adrenal fatigue, difficulty absorbing nutrients or a poor quality diet, dehydration, pregnancy (which can also cause hypertension), bed rest, consumption of alcohol, underactive thyroid, parathyroid disease, low blood sugar, and anemia. Low blood pressure often causes dizziness and fatigue. Spiritually, dizziness is about not feeling in control, feeling like you don't have a direction or purpose, and lack of organization.

IMMUNE SYSTEM
Chakras 7, 1, and Those Related to the Organs Impacted

There are many things that we can do to strengthen and protect our immune systems, such as the following:

- Eliminate as many chemicals from our water, food, environment, clothing, cleaning products, and personal products as possible.

- Heal the root causes of preexisting conditions, don't just band-aid symptoms.

- Support the health of our adrenal glands, since overactive adrenals produce too much cortisol. Cortisol and other steroid hormones are both anti-inflammatories and immune system suppressors, which is why steroids are often given for severe inflammation.

- Eat healthily, such as avoiding processed foods, inflammatory foods like sugar, excess gluten and dairy, and chemical-laden foods. Most of your diet should be fruits and vegetables, and we need to be sure to get enough complete proteins, healthy fats, and fiber.

- Reduce stress.

- Exercise.

- Be authentic and listen to intuition.

- Wash hands with nontoxic soap and wear a mask around people who may be unhealthy or possible carriers of disease.

- Express feelings and stand up for yourself.

- Reduce inflammation in the body.

- Avoid steroids and other medications that reduce immune system health, especially many medications for autoimmune diseases.

- Get enough rest and adequate sleep.

- Address gut-health issues. Most of one's immune system is contained in the gut. If you need to take antibiotics or other medications that may disrupt the bacterial balance or compromise the health of the stomach or intestinal lining, it can be very helpful to take probiotics and eat/drink fermented foods and beverages.

- Spend time with loved ones, including pets.
- Avoid negative people and situations that create negative energy.
- Express your creativity.
- Follow a spiritual practice.

Since the immune system is spiritually related to protection, if you are having issues with it, consider how you feel about your own physical and emotional safety. As I have said, one of the underlying issues concerning anxiety is not feeling safe. Healing from anxiety is important for many reasons, one of which is that anxiety causes the adrenal glands to produce too much cortisol. It becomes a vicious cycle.

If you do not feel safe and protected, it may stem from a childhood with parents or circumstances that did not provide emotional and physical protection. It may stem from being in an abusive relationship or not having a support system. It can be the result of being in a job that doesn't feel secure and that you may be at high risk of losing. Explore what aspects of your life, current and in the past, may be contributing to a lack of security, and take steps to address them, either through therapy, meditation (especially mindfulness work), spiritual grounding by being in nature, and through movement. Be honest with yourself about what you need to do to make things better, and work on finding a new job or going back to school, creating a new support system for yourself, or letting go of relationships that are no longer serving you.

INFLAMMATION
Chakras 7, 1, and Those Related to the Parts of the Body
Impacted

Inflammation is the body's natural response to injury, infection, or illness. It is also created as part of building and stretching healthy muscles. It has protective properties, but when it becomes chronic or excessive, it results in disease, pain, and even mental illness. Eating anti-inflammatory foods and increasing antioxidants can treat inflammation, as can exercise, stress reduction, mindfulness meditation, and certain homeopathic, nutritional, and herbal treatments tailored to the individual situation. Obesity, chronic stress, certain medications, sugar, refined carbs, trans fats, dairy, processed meat, and excessive alcohol can create inflammation. Other contributors to inflammation include toxins like mold, pollutants and smoking, gut imbalance, lack of movement, lack of sleep, and working out too much or too aggressively.

Since inflammation is linked to so many disease states and conditions, every effort should be made to treat and prevent it. The use of anti-inflammatory medications like ibuprofen can cause a rebound effect if used too often.

Spiritually, inflammation is about the swelling up of emotions, both positive and "negative." It is important to be able to both feel your emotions and express them appropriately.

KNEE PROBLEMS
Chakra 1

Spiritually, knees are about bending and being flexible. This may also pertain to trying to control your life moving forward or being open to change and suggestions. Having strong quadriceps, calves, and hamstrings and working on stretching and flexibility can help treat and prevent knee injuries. In the resources section of the appendix, there is a link with ten exercises to help heal knees. Certified trainers, physical therapists, or chiropractors are great sources of information for exercises and for learning how to properly align your hips, legs, and feet while walking. Often, we aren't even aware that we are not walking or standing straight.

LEARNING DISABILITIES
Chakras 7, 6, 3, and Those of Specific Body Parts Involved

It is important to identify learning disabilities using testing with a professional. Many people are not aware that most schools are required to test children for learning disabilities and other issues, at no charge, if a parent requests it. Suggested remedies include nontoxic living, reducing sugar and processed foods, looking for underlying issues such as Lyme disease, gut imbalance, and vision or hearing problems. Specific training and therapy with someone experienced in learning disabilities and learning styles can also be very helpful.

Spiritually it is helpful to look at the functions impacted by the disability. Difficulty with directions and spatial ability might indicate that the person is fearful of leaving home or venturing out. Dyslexia, or reversal of letters and words, might be indicative of someone who is overwhelmed by learning new things or maturing.

LIVER
Chakras 3, 6

I know a person who reversed his need for a liver transplant primarily by changing his outlook on life. Of course, he had stopped drinking alcohol and had begun to take vitamins, but it was by letting go of resentment and realizing that his family needed him that he was able to stop all medications and treatment and actually reverse a substantial amount of the damage to his liver, which doctors had said wasn't possible. His blood markers for liver disease have been in the normal, healthy range for the past twelve years.

Natural remedies to help strengthen the liver include omega-3s, coffee and green tea, eliminating chemicals and other toxins, exercise and maintenance of a healthy weight, and milk thistle. Avoid the use of Tylenol, sugar, and non-nutritious carbs. Burdock, berries, grapefruit, and garlic are helpful, as is aloe vera juice. It is also important to check for the blood disorder hemochromatosis and to check ferritin (iron storage) levels. Working with a homeopath or other natural practitioner can be a great source of alternative remedies and gentle cleanses. Harsh cleanses aren't necessary.

The liver is the seat of anger in Chinese medicine, and it is a part of the body that helps to process waste and toxins. Spiritually, be aware of the toxic feelings you are holding and the toxic people in your life. Do you feel like you are using your time productively and giving it to people who appreciate it, or do you feel like you are wasting it?

LYME DISEASE AND COINFECTIONS
Potentially All of the Chakras, Depending on the Parts of the Body Impacted

When a person comes to me needing help for "mystery symptoms," I have found that Lyme or Lyme coinfections are almost always involved. Many people don't realize that they have Lyme or Lyme coinfections because the symptoms mimic so many other conditions. Symptoms vary widely from case to case. A link to an extensive list created by the Global Lyme Alliance can be found in the resources section in the appendix. Even if clients have been tested, many of the results are false negatives so they don't get treatment. Often, only the Lyme bacteria *Borrelia burgdorferi* is tested for, so coinfections are missed.

Until 2019, the CDC only recognized two tests, the ELISA test and the Western blot, with the Western blot only given if the ELISA test is positive. It is widely recognized that the ELISA test is so inaccurate, due to its lack of sensitivity, that it gives false negatives about 50 percent of the time, and the Western blot isn't very respected by most knowledgeable Lyme practitioners, either. Neither test for coinfections. In 2019, the CDC finally cleared two tests that use sensitive enzyme immunoassay (EIA) techniques. I don't have much faith in any of these tests, unfortunately, and neither do many of the experienced practitioners I have worked with. There are other types of Lyme tests available, which are said to be more accurate but are unfortunately quite expensive. Unless a test is approved by the CDC, insurance companies will not pay for it.

Sadly, effective treatment is also lacking and can cause severe side effects. The Global Lyme Alliance lists more than one hundred potential symptoms of Lyme disease on their site, impacting virtually every part of the body. These symptoms can morph and change daily, making diagnosis and treatment even more difficult.

Studies have shown evidence that Lyme and related diseases can be transmitted by mosquitoes, spiders, large flies, and other insects including ticks. Lyme bacteria has been found in saliva, breast milk, urine, and other bodily fluids, such as semen and vaginal secretions. The jury is out about human-to-human transmission but many people, including myself, believe it is possible, and I know of entire families who are infected, including young children.

Viruses like EBV have been linked to Lyme disease in some cases, but they are separate entities. They may be found together but don't have to be. Viruses can make people more susceptible to getting Lyme disease because they weaken the immune system and may alter cells in a way that makes them more susceptible to bacterial or additional viral invaders. In 2015, Lyme, a chronic fatigue virus, and mold were detected in my body, but not EBV. I was told, and agreed, that I had likely contracted it as a young child growing up less than fifteen miles from Lyme, Connecticut, the town the disease was named after. After nine months of natural treatment, my symptoms were eradicated, along with symptoms I had not equated with Lyme, such as the depression I had battled since childhood. There has been no trace of Lyme discovered in me since that time.

Treatment Options

When I tell people that I am healed from Lyme and coinfections, the first thing I am asked is how I did it. It truly was a combination of physical, emotional, and spiritual "remedies" specifically designed for me by my treatment team and my intuition. While components of what worked for me would likely also help other people, I couldn't recommend the exact same "formulas" I used to effectively treat someone else. It is heartbreaking to hear about those who have been in physical and emotional pain for years, often unable to work, who have lost much of their support system, and who feel hopeless and helpless. I truly wish I could give easy, one-size-fits-all answers about healing, but I can't.

What I can do is to share what I know about healing from Lyme and some of the strategies that worked for me and many other people I have worked with directly or corresponded with.

- Using the intuitive writing technique, talk with your body, your symptoms, and the Lyme disease. Ask them the purpose of why you are sick and why it is using this to get your attention. With severe illness, the intuitive message is usually very important, along with the changes and challenges you are being asked to address. In my case, I knew I needed to write this book, but I was putting it off because I was afraid of being heard and seen and because I was afraid I couldn't do a good job.

- Follow the recommendations for autoimmune disease in that entry in this glossary.

- Antibiotics are the only FDA- (and insurance-) approved treatment for Lyme disease. From my research, experience, and information I receive from my guides, I have mixed feelings about them. They seem to be more effective at the onset of Lyme, when the symptoms first begin, and less effective for chronic Lyme or for people who discovered it after having symptoms for some time. I know of many, many people who received antibiotics after contracting the disease, with immediate symptom improvement, only to feel sick with the same or more severe symptoms months or even years later. Obviously, the antibiotics didn't eradicate the disease. I also know of people I have treated who became even more ill and close to losing their lives from high-dose, prolonged use of antibiotics. When the Lyme disease in my system was discovered, along with all of the tick-borne coinfections that commonly accompany Lyme, I vowed not to use antibiotics because I didn't believe in their effectiveness and because I have always had horrible physical and emotional side effects when taking them. I was fortunate to find a very experienced practitioner, a naturopath, who had been helping people heal from Lyme for decades, either without antibiotics or in some cases working in conjunction with another doctor who was treating patients with them.

- Test for, identify, and treat possible underlying and coexisting conditions. These may include mold exposure, viruses, parasites, other autoimmune conditions, or a compromised immune system. These conditions may be interfering with the body's natural ability to detox and to kill off the Lyme bacteria. I advise working with a practitioner who does not attempt to treat every condition at the same time. That is stressful for the body and makes it difficult to determine which treatments are effective or causing possible side effects.

- Gentle detoxing before beginning any treatment can cut down on the possible side effects of treatment. This helps to cleanse the system and put less stress on the immune system, liver, and lymphatic system later.

- Follow an anti-inflammatory diet, which includes avoiding gluten, dairy, sugar, and soy.

- Eliminate as many toxins and chemicals from your body and environment as possible to alleviate the stress placed on your immune system and organs that assist with detoxing, like the liver.

- Herbs, vitamins, and homeopathic remedies: There are many, many natural remedies that have been helpful in the treatment of Lyme, based on my experience, the experience of my clients, and others I regularly correspond with, including practitioners. These programs should be designed individually by experienced practitioners, based on the person's specific diseases, genetics, toxicity level and ability to detox, stress level, tolerance to the treatment, specific symptoms, financial situation, and support system. The formulations will vary over time, as the person responds. Everyone is different and every case of Lyme is different as well. I have never been enthusiastic about one-size-fits-all protocols or about people trying different remedies on their own, hoping that something will work. It is possible to do more harm than good.

- I know people who have had success with treatments such as ozone therapy, CBD and medical marijuana, and electronic frequency machines such as the Rife machine. Many of these are controversial and have not been widely tested scientifically. There have been studies showing evidence that marijuana and CBD are helpful in reducing pain and inflammation as well as helping with anxiety and insomnia.

You can find more information about Lyme disease in chapter 14 on the 1st chakra.

MENSTRUAL PROBLEMS AND PREMENSTRUAL SYNDROME
Chakras 2, 6

In addition to trauma related to sexual abuse or assault, I have also encountered menstrual difficulties in young women who are fearful of growing up, usually because of societal, cultural, or family responsibilities that they do not want or may not be ready for. Pressure to marry at a young age or to marry a person that has been arranged for you, an obligation to pursue a career your family approves of rather than following passions and interests, or fear of becoming just like a mother who is oppressed, abused, unhappy, or abusive herself can all manifest as physical symptoms.

Unfortunately, birth control that ceases menstruation, or antidepressants, have been the primary forms of treatment for menstrual problems, and these can cause serious side effects, especially long term. Mental health counseling, acupuncture, chiropractic treatment to check for hip alignment issues, and energy healing, like Reiki, Barbara Brennan healing, and Healing Touch (HT) are safe and effective alternatives to try before using medication.

NEUROLOGICAL DISORDERS, LIKE MS AND FIBROMYALGIA
Potentially All of the Chakras, Depending on the Parts of the Body Impacted

I know of many cases in which these diseases have been misdiagnosed and have turned out to be Lyme disease, mold exposure symptoms, and/or viruses like chronic fatigue or EBV. EBV is something many people, if not all people, have been exposed to at some point in their lives, just like many viruses, but exposure does not mean that these viruses are active or causing symptoms.

These types of diseases also benefit from emotional and spiritual attention, just as autoimmune diseases do. I don't believe that it is a coincidence that more women are stricken with autoimmune disease and things like MS and fibromyalgia, which cause disabling pain and difficulty with movement. Women often feel oppressed and powerless, unable to or not encouraged to use their voices and express their opinions. It has not been uncommon for me to find a correlation between these diseases and women who feel this way. When I have helped and encouraged them to be more assertive, find self-love, and become more comfortable with their own power, I have seen their symptoms decrease and even eventually dissipate.

Neurological disorders would also benefit from homeopathy, acupuncture and traditional Chinese medicine, anti-inflammatory and autoimmune diets, nontoxic living, working with an herbalist and/or naturopath, stress relief and meditation, and movement.

Spiritually, one should pay attention to individual symptoms. Autoimmune diseases are about attacking the self and not having self-love. Symptoms that prevent you from moving or walking may mean that you are afraid of moving forward in life and embracing love.

POLYCYSTIC OVARY SYNDROME (PCOS)
Chakras 7, 3, 2

PCOS can be difficult to diagnose, especially since there are no concrete tests for it. It is a common disorder that many women don't even realize they have. There are degrees of PCOS, like most other conditions, so each case tends to be different in severity and form. Often the ovarian cysts and follicles that surround the eggs are the least troubling of the symptoms and complications, which include the following:

- Pain and bloating in the abdomen
- Irregular periods, which may be infrequent or prolonged
- Excess androgens or male hormones, which result in acne, excess hair, and male pattern baldness
- Weight gain due to excess insulin and metabolic syndrome
- Sleep apnea
- Low-grade inflammation
- Infertility, miscarriage, or premature birth
- Gestational or type 2 diabetes
- Depression, anxiety, and eating disorders
- Cancer of the uterine lining

There is no cure for PCOS, but there are definitely things that can be done to reduce symptoms and improve quality of life, such as these:

- Maintain as healthy a weight as possible. You may gain weight more easily and it may be more difficult to lose, but obesity isn't necessarily a component of PCOS.
- Eat a plant-and-protein rich diet, reducing simple carbohydrates and especially sugar, which people who have insulin resistance and metabolic syndrome do not process well.
- Avoid chemicals and other toxins, especially those that mimic hormones.
- Exercise is very important.
- You may find it helpful to avoid inflammatory foods like gluten, dairy, and sugar.
- Get enough rest.

- Seek therapy for mood management and support with possible self-esteem issues.
- Medications like spironolactone, which reduce testosterone levels, can sometimes be helpful, but watch for complications, including excess potassium.
- Controlling ovulation using birth control can be helpful for preventing ovarian cysts, but these medications also come with serious side effects.
- Many professionals believe that PCOS "disappears" after menopause, with the ceasing of ovulation and lack of production of testosterone, but it is possible for symptoms like insulin resistance and metabolic syndrome to remain, usually to a lesser degree.

Spiritually, it is not uncommon for me to see women with PCOS who have issues with previous trauma, especially sexual abuse or assault, who do not feel empowered as women, or who have been part of families or workplaces where women aren't respected, who avoid intimacy, especially through sexual contact, and who are conflicted about having children or in difficult marriages. They also may be creative people who fear or avoid expressing their authentic selves using creative expression. Addressing these issues and working on healing can help with lessening of symptoms.

SEIZURES
Chakra 6

Natural remedies include CBD oil, ketogenic diet, vagus nerve stimulation, adequate rest and sleep, stress reduction, meditation, and grounding. Also investigate root causes, such as Lyme disease, brain tumors, and exposure to toxins.

When a person has a seizure, they neurologically disconnect from the rest of the world. I have worked with clients with seizures who are highly empathic and have psychic abilities. They often had people in their lives who were highly scientific or logical, who didn't believe in their abilities and weren't comfortable with them. Consequently, my clients tried to push down these abilities and not express them. Because psychic abilities are bridges between the conscious and unconscious world or between spiritual dimensions, they can be very powerful and have energetic properties of their own, and trying to suppress them is quite difficult.

I believe that suppressing these powerful abilities and energies creates a disturbance in the brain and body that causes a short circuit—thus a seizure.

One of my clients who had seizures as a young girl had persistent fears and beliefs that they were caused by a brain tumor. Her father happened to be a doctor, who thought she was being "dramatic and overly sensitive." Fortunately, her mother had some of the same psychic and empathic abilities, so she had a person to talk to openly.

She turned out to indeed have a brain tumor, which was diagnosed in her late teens. Removal of it has virtually stopped the seizures, and her father is now more open to what she has to say about spirituality, which has resulted in spiritual and personal growth throughout the entire family.

SINUS ISSUES, INCLUDING SINUS INFECTIONS
Chakras 6, 4, 1

The sinuses are about breath, the taking in of life. They are connected to the ears and eyes. If your sinuses are blocked, it is difficult to breathe life into your body and to hear and see well. Spiritually, sinus problems can be about wanting to shut out the world, using multiple senses.

Histamine intolerance can often come into play, so follow a

low-histamine diet and use the enzyme DAO (diamine oxidase) and other supplements that encourage antihistamine production in the body, like D-Hist and HistaBlock. Antihistamines made of chemicals can damage natural antihistamine production in the body, so you may want to avoid them. For a low-histamine diet, eliminate gluten, dairy, and other inflammatory foods. Hidden mold exposure and allergies can be contributing factors. Xlear is one of my favorite natural products; it is like a neti pot in a spray. Colloidal silver has been helpful for me for when I feel a sinus infection coming on. Place one drop of colloidal silver into each nostril while laying upside down, with your head hanging over the side of a bed or couch. Let each drop sit for a minute or two and sniff it in. Repeat several times throughout the day. Of course, always consult with a medical professional when needed.

Several different types of prescription and over-the-counter medications can contribute to histamine sensitivity, including anti-depressants, high blood pressure and heart rhythm drugs, muscle relaxants, narcotics, local anesthetics, and NSAIDS like ibuprofen. Certain strains of probiotics also promote histamines, such as *Lactobacillus casei, L. bulgaria, L. delbrueki,* and *L. helviticus* and *Streptococcus thermophilus*. Other strains, too numerous to mention, can help fight histamine production. At the end of the book, there is a recommendation for a product I use.

SKIN PROBLEMS
Chakras 7, 6, 3, 1

Spiritually, problems with the skin are about covering up emotions, fears, and insecurities. I have seen so many cases of skin conditions of all types improving and even healing once people allow themselves to first feel and then release their emotions in healthy and productive ways. Our skin is incredibly reactive to how we feel, and while we can hide our emotions, we can't hide our skin.

The location on the body is also important. For example, rashes or other skin conditions on the legs, which represent moving forward in life, might mean that you have anger, fear, or resentment about moving forward, and a rash on your vagina could be a way of pushing people, as well as intimacy, away. Pay attention to the chakra that corresponds with the location of the skin condition to understand what issues need to be addressed.

Physically, skin conditions commonly relate to hormones, allergies, sensitivities, or autoimmune conditions. Pay attention to when you have a reaction, when it becomes worse, and when it is improving. Make note of what you are eating, stressful situations, who else is present, what products you are using, and what you are thinking about, as well as where you are in your menstrual cycle, if you are female. Medications for skin conditions include steroids, antibody drugs, Accutane, and anti-inflammatories. All of these can cause serious and potentially dangerous side effects, so it is worth investigating natural treatments.

Hormone balancing, using supplements to reduce testosterone if you are producing too much, changing your diet—including eating unprocessed and less inflammatory foods—using organic and nontoxic products, addressing sensitivities, using nonsteroidal topical products, reducing stress, and practicing mindfulness meditation can positively impact skin-related symptoms. Dairy and chocolate may contribute to acne in some people.

SLEEP HABITS
Chakras 7, 6, 5, 4

Sleep is one of the most important ingredients for health and wellness. These are some helpful hints for healthy habits:

- Go to bed and wake up at the same time every day.

- Exercise: Some people are stimulated by movement at night so you might want to exercise earlier in the day.

- Reduce stress so you don't ruminate about stressors when you are trying to fall asleep.

- Meditate, especially before bed.

- Take melatonin, valerian root, and/or sleepy teas.

- Do not drink caffeine after noon.

- Sleep in a very dark room, limiting exposure to electronics for an hour before bedtime.

- Play white noise.

- Make sure the temperature in the room is comfortable and low enough.

- Replace your mattress and/or pillow if they are not supportive or comfortable.

- Support your adrenals with supplements like ashwagandha, rhodiola (herbs that help the body manage stress), and possibly DHEA, a hormone the body produces in the adrenal gland that helps your body make other hormones, including sex hormones. DHEA begins to decline in our early 30s. I suggest that people have their DHEA levels checked by their doctors before beginning this supplement because of side effects, such as acne and abnormal hair growth in women. It is not recommended in people with a risk of hormone-sensitive cancer. I also suggest that people have their levels of cortisol checked, which helps to determine the health of their adrenal glands. High levels of cortisol can cause insomnia or sleep disturbance.

- Have your hormones checked for hormone imbalance. This can happen at any age, not just related to menopause.

- Be sure you are eating enough and getting enough complete proteins for the amino acids needed to create neurochemicals that impact energy and the ability to relax.

- Try CBD oil.
- Take herbal remedies from traditional Chinese medicine.

STIFF NECK AND SHOULDERS
Chakra 5

When I paint someone with very wide shoulders during a reading, that is a sign not only of issues in this area, but also someone who symbolically has "the weight of the world on their shoulders." The neck and shoulders are very common areas to hold stress, especially in people who do not easily express their feelings. Movement and stretching are very important, as is paying attention to your posture even while sitting and especially while looking at phones and computers.

Shoulder and neck injuries are common, unfortunately, because these are areas that we don't often think to strengthen and may not have the opportunity to strengthen or keep flexible. Strengthening the lats and upper back can also be helpful in reducing shoulder and neck injuries and helping them to heal.

TINNITUS
Chakra 6

Traditional treatments such as tricyclic antidepressants (an older form of antidepressant used before SSRIs like Prozac) or Xanax have side effects and are not always effective. They work by increasing the amount of the calming brain transmitter GABA. There are nontoxic, natural ways to increase GABA as well, such as taking liposomal GABA (easier to absorb than traditional GABA can be) and using the amino acid L-glutamine and the herb ginkgo biloba. Tinnitus can be a symptom of Lyme disease if it accompanies other symptoms, so this is something to be aware of.

Spiritually, ear issues are connected to things we may not want to hear or to needing to listen more closely. Ask yourself if either or both of these factors may be playing a part in tinnitus, hearing loss, or other ear conditions.

ULCERS, *H. PYLORI* BACTERIA, AND THE GUT
Chakras 5, 3

Ulcers are sores on the lining of your stomach, small intestine, or throat. Most are located in the small intestine and are called duodenal ulcers. Stomach ulcers are called gastric ulcers. Ulcers in the throat are called esophageal ulcers. Approximately 10 percent of the population are afflicted.[26]

It used to be thought that ulcers were caused exclusively by stress, until it was discovered that one of two causes are the *Helicobacter pylori* (*H. pylori*) bacteria, which is found in about 50 percent of the world's population, often without symptoms. It can be transmitted from person to person. The other cause is pain-relieving NSAID medications, like ibuprofen, but certain conditions can make people more susceptible. These include liver, kidney, or lung disease, a family history, smoking, and regular alcohol consumption.[27]

Traditional therapy includes antibiotics and antacids, however you may find relief from the pain of a stomach ulcer as well as digestive and gut issues if you practice the following:[28]

- Choose a healthy diet. A diet full of fruits—especially with vitamins A and C— vegetables, and whole grains. Not eating vitamin-rich foods may make it difficult for your body to heal your ulcer.
- Consider foods containing probiotics. These include yogurt, aged cheeses, miso, and sauerkraut. You can also take probiotics as a supplement.

- Consider eliminating milk and dairy. Sometimes drinking milk will make your ulcer pain better but then later cause excess acid, which increases pain. Dairy is also inflammatory.

- Consider switching pain relievers; if you use NSAIDs, consider finding nonpharmaceutical methods for reducing pain.

- Control stress. Stress may worsen the signs and symptoms of a peptic ulcer. Consider the sources of your stress and do what you can to address the causes. Some stress is unavoidable, but you can learn to cope with stress by exercising, spending time with friends, or writing in a journal.

- Don't smoke. Smoking may interfere with the protective lining of the stomach, making your stomach more susceptible to the development of an ulcer. Smoking also increases stomach acid.

- Limit or avoid alcohol. Excessive use of alcohol can irritate and erode the mucous lining in your stomach and intestines, causing inflammation and bleeding.

- Try to get enough sleep. Sleep can help your immune system and therefore counter stress. Also, avoid eating shortly before bedtime.

- Flavonoids are compounds that occur naturally in many fruits and vegetables. Foods and drinks rich in flavonoids include: soybeans, legumes, red grapes, kale, broccoli, apples, berries, and green tea. These can help reduce the symptoms of ulcers and promote healing.

- Using probiotic strains that help eradicate *H. Pylori,* specifically *Lactobacillus, Saccharomyces boulardii, L. acidophilus,* and *Bifidobacterium lactis.*

- There is also some evidence that zinc can help heal ulcers.

- A number of botanicals are recommended for treating peptic ulcers, including turmeric, mastic, cabbage, deglycyrrhizinated licorice, and neem bark extract.

Spiritually, ulcers are about open wounds, emotional pain, unexpressed stress and resentment, and feeling oppressed. In addition to the 3rd chakra chapter for stomach and intestinal ulcers, it is helpful to look at the "Call to Action" items in the 5th chakra chapter as well, since the throat is the route of expression for feelings. Many people feel their own and other people's emotions in the gut area, so be sure to ask yourself if what you are feeling is your own emotions or if you are picking them up from other people around you. Setting proper boundaries is very important.

The gut (stomach and intestines) is a common location for pain and discomfort. According to the website www.gialliance .com, more Americans are hospitalized for digestive-related diseases than any other condition and nearly twenty million Americans have chronic digestive conditions. I suspect that the number is even higher because many people I have encountered, including myself, don't even think to report things like bloating, nausea, digestive issues related to menstruation, motion sickness, constipation, and food sensitivities to their physician. After trying countless natural remedies, medications, lifestyle changes, and therapies without success or being told that the issue is "in their head," they give up trying to feel better and just "learn to live with it."

Discovering the root cause(s) can be very challenging and traditional tests like an upper or lower GI series, when barium is ingested during an X-ray, using a camera to look inside the digestive tract, barium enemas, colonoscopy, or endoscopic ultrasound often do not provide answers. Stool sampling, usually offered by alternative or integrative physicians more than traditional practitioners, may be useful to help find parasites or bacterial imbalances. Food allergies or sensitivities can be the culprits but are tricky to diagnose. Please see the section on food allergies and sensitivities earlier in this glossary for more information.

In my experience, there are usually multiple root causes

for gut disorders: a combination of physical, environmental, emotional, and spiritual issues. Gut disorders can be hereditary as well. Not only physically as in the case of autoimmune diseases like Crohn's but emotionally as well. I have commonly encountered unexplained gut issues in families going back several generations. I believe that we all have "vulnerable areas" that tend to react more intensely to physical or emotional stress than other areas of the body. I have had gut issues for as long as I can remember like many members of my family. Avoiding gluten and dairy, taking steps to avoid constipation, using digestive enzymes, and stress release has helped tremendously but has not eliminated the symptoms entirely. Please refer to the chapter about the 3rd chakra for more information about gut and digestive issues.

VIRUSES
Chakras 7, 1, and the Areas of the Body Impacted

Epstein-Barr virus, or EBV, is not a new phenomenon. It was first discovered over forty-five years ago in cells isolated from African Burkitt lymphoma, and it has been studied ever since. It can be transmitted orally, through blood transfusion, and by organ implantation. It is a member of the herpes virus family, most commonly associated with and the cause of mononucleosis. It is estimated that antibodies for EBV can be detected in 90 percent of the population, usually as a result of childhood infection.

I have read claims by some people that latent viruses, especially Epstein-Barr, are the root causes of Lyme disease, fibromyalgia, other autoimmune conditions, and cancer. Using the term "cause" is deceiving. Viruses themselves can cause autoimmune symptoms. Research is being conducted to investigate the possibility that various viruses may trigger specific autoimmune diseases in people already at risk, possibly genetically or with a latent condition. I have worked with many people, including myself, with Lyme disease but no trace of EBV in their bodies.

Having certain viruses, especially EBV, just like mold or other toxicity, chemical exposure, stress, or any number of other things, can make us more *susceptible* to disease. Anything that creates stress or toxicity puts a strain on our immune systems and can increase our chances of contracting disease, including cancer.

EBV can be latent, active, or chronic. The reactivation and mutation of certain strains of EBV has been linked to some rare forms of cancer, since mutations in cells infected with EBV can lead to cancerous changes, and initial studies have found a possible genetic-environmental link between EBV and lupus, multiple sclerosis, rheumatoid arthritis, inflammatory bowel disease, type 1 diabetes, juvenile idiopathic arthritis, and celiac disease, potentially signifying that having EBV puts one at greater risk of developing these diseases.[29] There may also be a link between schizophrenia and EBV. In a study of 700 people, all with EBV but with and without schizophrenia found that participants with genetic risk factors for schizophrenia as well as elevated antibodies for EBV were over eight times more likely to have schizophrenia than the control group.[30] With over 90 percent of the population having contracted EBV and likely 100 percent of the population exposed to it, proving a direct causal relationship is challenging.

In rare cases, EBV can lead to a chronic condition called CAEBV, and it is diagnosed using symptoms and a blood test showing chronic active infection. The only recognized treatment for the active form is stem-cell transplant, but I know of clients who are being treated for and improving from symptoms of what appears to be latent EBV. There is controversy over whether latent EBV can cause symptoms and whether or not the latent form is truly latent.

What does all of this mean for you? If you suspect or wonder about EBV or other types of viruses, in my experience you may find more help with diagnosis and possible treatment using an alternative practitioner like a naturopath or integrative physician. You may find them to be more open and more informed about the subject. As with all viruses, you can benefit from an autoimmune, anti-inflammatory diet, natural ways to improve your immune system, connection to intuition, stress reduction, and supplements, including homeopathy, which should be individualized depending on your symptoms and specific condition.

Spiritually, viruses can be about a sense of fear or dread, difficulty creating healthy boundaries, and not taking time to rest or otherwise take care of yourself. Individual symptoms should also be considered when determining spiritual root causes, such as chronic EVB or a chronic fatigue virus, where someone may not be owning their own power and feel vulnerable because they were not able to put the virus into remission.

VISION PROBLEMS
Chakra 6

Several vitamins and herbs have been shown effective in preventing vision problems. These include the following:

- Bilberry
- Ginkgo biloba
- Saint-John's-wort
- Eyebright
- Zinc
- Lutein
- Vitamins A, E, and C
- Other antioxidants
- Omega-3 and omega-6 fatty acids

Always wear sunglasses with UV protection. Many people live with dry eyes and don't even realize it. As an alternative to eye drops, you can have plugs implanted painlessly into your tear ducts, which many insurances pay for. Wearing an eye mask while you sleep can reduce moisture loss, especially if you use a ceiling fan. Limit screen time and protect against blue light.

Spiritually, vision issues are related to what you don't want to see or what you aren't paying attention to.

Epilogue

How to Use This Book Going Forward

We continue to learn, grow, and change until the day we are no longer on this earth and, I believe, even as we transform into pure energy, leaving our bodies behind. If we let fear get in the way of that growth, life becomes stagnant and unfulfilling. Fear dampens communication with Spirit and our intuition. A life dominated by fear, without happiness and purpose, often contributes to physical, emotional, and spiritual illness.

Even highly spiritual people, who have been on a conscious spiritual and health journey for many decades, need to continue to challenge themselves and expand their potential for healing and growth. We are always discovering parts of our personalities and behaviors that can be adjusted to assist in our growth and wellness as well as our strengths and abilities. Hopefully, we never stop learning deeper ways to love and accept ourselves. We are always works in progress, and that is okay. It is also important to do all of this at our own pace and allow for mistakes along the way.

The tools in this book are designed to be used throughout

your entire lifetime. If you are a practitioner, you can use them to help others. If you are a parent, I encourage you to use what you have learned in the book to help your children, especially to connect with their intuition.

I suggest creating a new intuitive painting at least every six months, along with checking in with your intuition and the chakra chart you created to see what has changed, the progress you have made, and any obstacles you have encountered. You may discover additional issues and strengths as well as additional root causes. You may decide that the strategies and tools you initially chose aren't working and that others fit better with your lifestyle and beliefs. Keep an open mind. If doing this every six months seems overwhelming, perhaps once a year is more appropriate. You can also make an individual appointment with me for a reading and to evaluate the progress you have made on your own. My website is www.katiebeecher.com.

Please feel free to contact me on social media and email to let me know how you are personally using the book and to tell me your stories.

ACKNOWLEDGMENTS

With Love and Gratitude

To my family—Brad, Lauren, Larissa, Corey, and Thomas: I can never express the amount of gratitude and love I feel for you. Thank you for your endless support and encouragement. You never let me give up and you are my greatest cheerleaders. Thank you for your hours (days) of reading and editing.

To Walter and Mary Taras, my incredible grandparents, for their unconditional love and acceptance.

To Jean Sutherland, MSW, my very first therapist. Thank you for saving my life, helping me recover, and teaching me about Jungian psychology. Thanks to Jungian therapist Nora Dixon, who helped me through some very dark times.

To my literary agent, Ellen Scordato, to Alison Fargis, and everyone at Stonesong, and to Joel Fotinos, Gwen Hawkes, and everyone at St. Martin's Press and Macmillan Publishers: I am so very grateful for your belief in me, my message, and the work that I do. Thank you for the advice, editing, and positivity. I look forward to our continued work together.

To God and my guides for my amazing intuitive and medium abilities and your unconditional love.

To my friends, clients, and followers on social media. Thank you for allowing me into your lives, trusting me with your precious secrets, and for being part of your healing journeys. I so appreciate your support, valuable comments, and belief in me and the work that I do.

To my friend Catherine Glastal. You generously invited me to New Jersey and helped me grow my business, then connected me with Stonesong Literary Agency. I am so grateful for the support and friendship I found in Westfield and can't wait to visit again.

To all of my readers and editors, including my dear friends Aubrey Graf-Daniels and Linda Tavares. I truly appreciate your time, advice, and endless support. Thanks to Cherise Fisher for helping me write my proposal and for encouraging me to always be true to myself.

To my pole family at Bittersweet Studios in Jacksonville, Florida. Love you all.

APPENDIX

Websites, Resources, Healing Therapies, and Recommended Products

The following section contains additional information about reference tools, resources, and treatments I have referred to in the book, used myself, or that have been recommended by others. This is not an exhaustive list of the types of quality treatments and healing modalities available. I am an affiliate of several of these companies, which are followed by an asterisk. I am extremely selective about the products and companies I endorse, and I do not do so unless I have personally used them and found them to be effective and of the highest quality.

FAVORITE WEBSITES

Environmental Working Group. www.ewg.org: Information about nontoxic products and safe, organic food.

National Resources Defense Council. www.nrdc.org. Environmental action group.

Knee exercises. https://www.healthline.com/health/exercises-for -knee-pain#strengthening-exercises.

Cynthia Li, MD, who wrote about her personal healing journey from autoimmune disease. www.cynthialimd.com.

Surviving Mold. www.survivingmold.com: Resources on toxic mold and how to treat the symptoms associated with exposure to it.

National Vaccine Information Center. www.nvic.org: Information about vaccine safety and laws.

Stink! (2015) A documentary directed by Jon Whelan, available on Netflix, about the toxicity of artificial fragrances.

American Association of Naturopathic Physicians. www.naturopathic .org/medicine.

Mary Coyle, homeopath extraordinaire. www.realchildcenter.com.

Helping mood disorders using food and supplements. Julia Ross's book *The Mood Cure* (Penguin Life, 2003) is an excellent resource. https://www.juliarosscures.com/mood-cure/.

The Body Keeps the Score (Penguin Books, 2003) is an essential read for anyone interested in trauma and its impact on the body. https:// www.besselvanderkolk.com/resources/the-body-keeps-the-score.

A website and group of books by Dr. Elaine Aron about highly sensitive and empathic people. She was one of the first to write about this subject. https://hsperson.com/.

Information about the personality typology test based on Jungian theories about how we view the world. www.myersbriggs.org.

Information about Carl Jung. https://www.cgjungpage.org/.

LYME DISEASE RESOURCES

Bay Area Lyme—useful information about Lyme disease: www .bayarealyme.org.

A list of Lyme disease symptoms. https://globallymealliance.org/wp -content/uploads/2019/11/Lyme-disease-symptoms_GLA_1119 .pdf.

There are numerous Lyme disease accounts on social media that are excellent sources of resources, information, and support.

ENERGY HEALING AND OTHER HEALING THERAPIES

HEALING TOUCH

Founded by registered nurse Janet Mentgen in 1989, Healing Touch (HT) is an energy therapy in which practitioners consciously use their hands and intent to promote health and healing. HT utilizes only very light or near-body touch to influence the energy field that penetrates and surrounds the body. Many types of energy medicine employ techniques to influence these fields by applying light or near-body touch on the body or by placing the hands in or through the field. Qigong, Jin Shin Jyutsu, and Reiki are other examples of this type of therapeutic approach. www.healingtouchprogram.com.

SHIATSU

Shiatsu is based on pressure points similar to the points used in acupuncture or reflexology. It is performed using the fingers, although certain devices may also be used. Shiatsu works on the theory that the human body has energy centers that are interconnected by energy channels, or meridians. https://zensomamassage.com/shiatsu-energy-balancing-for-health-and-wellness/.

REIKI

Reiki is an ancient Japanese technique for hands on healing. reiki.org.

BARBARA BRENNAN SCHOOL OF HEALING

In 1982, Barbara Brennan, a former NASA physicist, founded the Barbara Brennan School of Healing. She devised a series of intuitive energy healing techniques that involve clearing, energetic balancing, and renewal. barbarabrennan.com.

CRANIOSACRAL THERAPY

Craniosacral therapy, also called cranial osteopathy and cranial therapy, is a manual, noninvasive therapy using gentle hand pressure to manipulate the skeleton and connective tissues, typically the head, skull, and sacrum (the large triangular bone at the base of the spinal column). It releases tensions in the body for pain relief and improves immune system function and overall health. https://www.drweil .com/health-wellness/balanced-living/wellness-therapies/cranial -osteopathy/.

KUNDALINI YOGA

I love Kundalini yoga for so many reasons. It is a type of yoga that helps us connect to our intuition and our bodies using movement, chanting, and meditation designed for specific parts of the body, conditions, and chakras. It is physically, emotionally, and spiritually therapeutic. www.3HO.org; www.kundaliniyoga.org.

BODY CODE/EMOTION CODE

Body Code and Emotion Code are techniques for gathering information and balancing the body. I have had this done and found it helpful. https://discoverhealing.com/the-body-code/.

LYMPHATIC MASSAGE

Lymphatic drainage is a form of massage that stimulates the movement of lymph fluids around the body. There are machines that help lymphatic fluid drainage also. This helps remove waste and toxins from the bodily tissues. Some health conditions can benefit from lymphatic massage, include lymphedema, fibromyalgia, skin disorders, edema, hormone imbalance, digestive disorders, fatigue, and insomnia.

RECOMMENDED PRODUCTS

CBD oil: My favorite is made by Remedy Plant Lab,* www .remedyplantlab.com. I received a sample of the vanilla avocado oil, and my husband and I have both been using it to help us sleep and for pain relief. We call it our magic oil because it works! Pain my husband experienced for over ten years from surgery to remove a joint in his toe is not only gone, but he has more flexibility as well, and I'm sleeping better than ever. For a 10 percent discount, use the code Katie10.

Supplement gummies: www.maryruthorganics.com.

Vitamix: www.vitamix.com. The blender I use for my smoothies and also for juicing.

Home laser: Nira skin.* Have found this helpful for softening fine lines and scars, www.niraskin.com. For 10 percent off, use the code Katie10.

Hair testing for vitamins and minerals along with nutritional advice: Sassy Holistics, www.sassyholistics.com.

Oracle cards: Keepers of the Light, Animal Medicine Cards.

NATURAL PERSONAL AND BEAUTY PRODUCTS

Natural beauty and skin care by Miranda Kerr: www.koraorganics .com

www.badgerbalm.com

https://ctorganics.com/

www.beechersbotanicals.com

https://labrunaskincare.com/

https://www.briutessentials.com/

https://www.tomsofmaine.com/

https://lordjones.com/

www.aveda.com

www.cygallebeauty.com

www.burtsbees.com

www.follain.com.

Natural tick repellent: www.ticktocknaturals.com

GLUTEN-FREE FOOD BRANDS

Amy's foods even has candy bars and they are delicious. www.amys
.com

Hu Kitchen offers amazing chocolate and gluten-free crackers. For
15 percent off, use the code KatieBeecher15. www.hukitchen.com*

Probiotics: www.justthrivehealth.com.* For 15 percent off, use the
code Beecher15. These are also histamine free.

SUPPLEMENT CREAMS

My favorites are by Radiate Wellness: https://www.radiatewellness
products.com/.* They make a wide variety of effective creams (I have
tried the majority), ranging from natural estrogen and progesterone,
DHEA, to natural ingredients to increase energy and sex drive, magnesium, and B vitamins.

NOTES

1. https://www.sciencedaily.com/releases/2019/06/190627113951
   .htm.
2. https://www.healthline.com/health/what-is-dmt#presence
   -in-brain.
3. https://www.ncbi.nlm.nih.gov/pmc/articles/PMC4740614/.
4. www.avoicefortheinnocent.org.
5. www.RAINN.org.
6. https://ghr.nlm.nih.gov/primer/howgeneswork/epigenome.
7. https://www.sciencemag.org/news/2019/07/parents-emotional
   -trauma-may-change-their-children-s-biology-studies-mice
   -show-how.
8. www.Adultchildren.org.
9. https://www.naturalmedicinejournal.com/journal/2017–10
   /current-controversy-does-adrenal-fatigue-exist.
10. https://www.aaaai.org/conditions-and-treatments/asthma.
11. https://www.ncbi.nlm.nih.gov/pmc/articles/PMC7053252
    /#:~:text=Caffeine%20appears%20to%20improve%20airways,
    -cause%20misinterpretation%20of%20the%20results.
12. https://pubmed.ncbi.nlm.nih.gov/10724294/#:~:text=Significant
    %20data%20suggest%20that%20hypnosis,randomized%2C%20
    controlled%20studies%20are%20needed.

13. https://www.ncbi.nlm.nih.gov/pmc/articles/PMC4391363/.
14. https://www.nutritics.com/p/news_Why-Most-Iron-In-Spinach-Is-Useless#:~:text=Studies%20have%20shown%20that%20as,is%20around%2015%20%2D35%25.
15. https://www.bones.nih.gov/health-info/bone/osteoporosis/overview Osteoporosis.
16. https://www.nof.org/.
17. https://www.ncbi.nlm.nih.gov/pmc/articles/PMC3018605/#:~:text=Cardiovascular%20dis ease%20develops%207%20to%2010%20years%20later%20in%20women,'protected'%20against%20cardio vascular%20disease.
18. https://www.raynauds.org/.
19. https://www.diabetes.org/.
20. https://www.ncbi.nlm.nih.gov/pmc/articles/PMC2570378/.
21. https://www.mayoclinic.org/diseases-conditions/diabetes/symptoms-causes/syc-20371444.
22. https://repository.up.ac.za/handle/2263/44393 https://journals.lww.com/co-obgyn/Abstract/2016/06000/The_impact_of_stress_on_fertility_treatment.10.aspx.
23. https://readysetfood.com/blogs/community/food-allergies-in-children-v-adults.
24. https://www.foodallergy.org/resources/facts-and-statistics; https://medalerthelp.org/blog/allergy-statistics/#food-allergy.
25. https://www.cnbc.com/2016/09/09/allergies-are-on-the-rise-and-here-are-three-reasons-why.html.
26. https://familydoctor.org/condition/ulcers/.
27. https://www.mayoclinic.org/diseases-conditions/peptic-ulcer/diagnosis-treatment/drc-20354229.
28. https://my.clevelandclinic.org/health/diseases/10350-peptic-ulcer-disease/prevention.
29. https://www.ncbi.nlm.nih.gov/pmc/articles/PMC6008310/#B4.
30. https://academic.oup.com/schizophreniabulletin/article/45/5/1112/5193713.

INDEX

abandonment, 61, 113, 119, 133, 182, 185
acid rebound, 197
acid reflux, 196–98
   5th Chakra and, *113,* 126, 127, 155
   case study, Claire, 155, 157
acupuncture, 211
   for addictions, 202
   for ADHD, 200
   for adrenal glands, 204
   for asthma, 211
   for back pain, 214
   for cardiovascular disease, 222
   connecting to intuition through, 53
   detoxing, 96, 97
   for gallbladder, 238
   for gut health, 142
   for headaches, 239
   for menstrual problems, 253
   for neurological disorders, 254
   resources, 275
addiction, 201–2
   1st Chakra and, 176, *176*
   3rd Chakra and, 142, 143
   6th Chakra and, 94
   7th Chakra, 83, *83*
   depression and, 206
   dysfunctional family member and, 185–86

personal chakra issue checklist, 65
ADHD/ADD, 198–201
adrenal fatigue, 117, *141,* 171, 203–5, 243
adrenal glands, 203–5
   4th Chakra and, 131
   5th Chakra and, 115
   anxiety and depression, 207
   blood pressure and, 243
   chronic fatigue syndrome and, 223
   detoxing, 96
   immune system and, 244
   weight loss and, 147
adrenaline, 183, 201, 227
Adult Children of Alcoholics (ACOA), 127, 143, 157, 182–84, 187, 202
affirmations
   1st Chakra, 178
   2nd Chakra, 162
   3rd Chakra, 144
   4th Chakra, 132
   5th Chakra, 116
   6th Chakra, 98
   7th Chakra, 85
AIDS, *176*
Ajna. See Chakra, 6th

alcohol
  1st Chakra and, 177
  4th Chakra and, 131
  anxiety and depression, 207
  bones and, 217, 218
  heart disease and blood pressure,
    221, 243
  inflammation and, 246
  ulcers and, 262, 263
alcoholism, 70, 73, 104, 127, 143, 155,
    156, 157, 181–84, 189, 201–2
  PTSD and, 164
  sexual abuse or assault, 167
allergies, 96, 208–9, 239, 258, 259
  food, 95, 235–37, 264
alopecia, 212
Anahata. See Chakra, 4th
anemia, 215, 253, 256
anger, 49, 55, 97, 168, 185, 248
anorexia nervosa, 149–50, 197
antacids, 196–97, 262
antibiotics, 64, 196, 235, 244, 251, 262
antidepressants, 22, 152–53, 207,
    253, 261
antihistamines, 258
anti-inflammatories, 65, 259
anti-inflammatory diet. *See* diet
antioxidants, 210, 212, 246, 267
anxiety, 13–14, 205–8
  4th Chakra and, 130
  6th Chakra and, 94, 104
  addiction and, 201–2
  chronic fatigue syndrome and, 223
  headaches and, 239
  as obstacle to connecting with
    intuition, 40
  personal chakra issue checklist, 63
  treatment options, 206–8
Armour Thyroid, 65, 118
art therapy exercise, for body
    dysmorphia, 153–54
asthma, 208–11
  4th Chakra and, *130*
  case study, Claire, 156
  risk factors, 209
  symptoms of, 208–9
  treatment options, 209–11
"aura," 34
authenticity, 64, 87, 94, 103, 115, 121,
    161, 244

autism, 46–47, 199
autoimmune diet, 115, 117–18, 254
autoimmune diseases, 211–13,
    225–26. *See also specific diseases*
  1st Chakra and, 176, *176*, 177
  5th Chakra and, *113*, 115, 116–17
  6th Chakra and, 105
  anxiety and depression, 206
  diet for, 230–31
ayahuasca, 93

backaches (back pain), 70, *160*, 168,
    213–14
Barrett's Esophagus, 197
benzophenone, 118
bilberry, 267
binge eating (bingeing), 150
  author's story, 21, 22, 37, 66
biotin, 242
birth control, 215, 253, 256
bladder, 214–15
bloating, 236, 255, 264
blood diseases, 215–17
blood pressure, 215–16
  high. *See* high blood pressure
  low. *See* low blood pressure
blood sugar, 79, 200, 204, 223, 225–30
  symptoms of low, 226–27
blue color, *49*, 112
blurred/impaired vision, 104, 227
body disconnection, and 7th Chakra,
    83, *83*
body image, 22, 40, *141*, 145–49
  2nd Chakra and, 159–60
  3rd Chakra and, 140–41, *141*, 142
  addressing issues about food and,
    152–55
  personal chakra issue checklist, 63
bone density, 176, *176*, 177, 217–18,
    219, 241
bones, 217–19
  1st Chakra and, 61, *76*
boredom, 199, 224
boswellia, 213
boundaries, setting, 63–64, 133, 186–87
brain fog, 204
breast cancer, 136, 219–20, 219–21
breast feeding, 212, 235
breasts, *130*, 165–66
breast self-exams, 131

breathing, 131, 204, 210
bulimia, 150
    author's story, 1, 2, 13, 19–20,
        23–24, 56–57, 119, 146
bullying, 165–67

caffeine, 200, 204, 206, 207, 210, 223,
    229, 260
Call to Action, 11, 79–81, 195
    1st Chakra, 177–78
    2nd Chakra, 161–62
    3rd Chakra, 143–44
    4th Chakra, 131–32
    5th Chakra, 114–15
    6th Chakra, 95–97
    7th Chakra, 84
Campbell, Joseph, 55
cardiovascular disease, 60, *130,* 136,
    177, 221–22
career decisions, 61, 160, 233
    personal chakra issue checklist,
        63, 66
CBD oil, 252, 256, 261, 277
celiac disease, 212, 213, 218, 236, 266
cesarean deliveries, 209, 235
chakras
    overview of, 29–30
    use of term, 10
Chakra, 1st (root), 10, 29, *30,* 175–91
    affirmations, 178
    Call to Action, 177–78
    case study, Sheila, 187–90
    condition spotlight, 179–87
    Intuitive Writing Prompts, 177
    Mary's chakra chart, 72–73
    root causes for issues, 176, *176*
    sample charts, *34, 76*
    visualizations, 178
Chakra, 2nd (sacral), 29, *30,* 159–74
    affirmations, 162
    Call to Action, 161–62
    case study, Jill, 171–73
    condition spotlight, 163–71
    Intuitive Writing Prompts, 161
    Mary's chakra chart, 72
    root causes for issues, 160, *160*
    sample charts, *33, 76*
    visualizations, 162
Chakra, 3rd (solar plexus), 29, *30,*
    140–58

affirmations, 144
    Call to Action, 143–44
    case study, Claire, 155–57
    condition spotlight, 145–55
    Intuitive Writing Prompts, 143
    Mary's chakra chart, 72
    root causes for issues, *141,* 141–42
    sample charts, *33, 75*
    visualizations, 144
Chakra, 4th (heart), 29, *30,* 129–39
    affirmations, 132
    Call to Action, 131–32
    case study, Caroline, 136–38
    condition spotlight, 133–36
    Intuitive Writing Prompts, 130–31
    Mary's chakra chart, 72
    root causes for issues, 130, *130*
    sample charts, *32, 75*
    visualizations, 132
Chakra, 5th (throat), 29, *30,* 112–28
    affirmations, 116
    Call to Action, 114–15
    case study, Derek, 126–27
    condition spotlight, 116–25
    Intuitive Writing Prompts, 114
    Mary's chakra chart, 71–72
    root causes for issues, *113,* 113–14
    sample charts, *32, 75*
    visualizations, 116
Chakra, 6th (third eye), 29, *30,*
    92–111
    affirmations, 98
    Call to Action, 95–97
    case study, "Amy," 104–6
    condition spotlight, 98–103
    Intuitive Writing Prompts, 95
    Mary's chakra chart, 71
    root causes for issues, *93,* 94–95
    sample charts, *31, 74*
    visualizations, 98
Chakra, 7th (crown), 10–11, 29, *30,*
    82–91
    affirmations, 85
    Call to Action, 84
    condition spotlight, 85–91
    Intuitive Writing Prompts,
        83–84
    Lyme disease and, 56–57
    Mary's chakra chart, 71
    root causes for issues, 83, *83*

Chakra, 7th (crown) (cont'd)
  sample charts, *31, 74*
  visualizations, 85
chakra chart worksheet, 291–92
  personal chakra issue checklist,
    62–67
  practice case study, Mary, 69–73
  sample charts, *31–34, 74–76*
chi (qi), 30, 57
chiropracty, 210, 214, 239, 247, 253
chronic dieting, 143, 145–49
chronic fatigue syndrome, 222–24, 234
circadian rhythms, 92
cleanliness and "hygiene hypothesis,"
    235
clumsiness, 227
coenzyme Q-10 (CoQ10), 222
coffee, 198, 210, 248
coffee enemas, 64, 96
cognitive behavioral therapy, 170,
    202
cold feet and/or hands, 224–25
colostrum, 212
connecting to intuition, 3–4, 10, 13,
    23, 37–54, 78, 102, 119
  obstacles to, 38–42
  quiz about intuitive and psychic
    skills, 106–9
  symptoms as messages, 55–58
  technique one: Written Dialogue,
    42–45
  technique two: Intuitive Soul
    Painting, 45–49
  technique three: dream
    interpretation, 50–51
  technique four: oracle cards,
    pendulums, and runes, 51–53
  tips for increasing, 109–10
coordination problems, 227
corticosteroids, 209–10, 218
cortisol, 60, *141,* 147, 203–4, 244,
    245, 260
Coxsackievirus B (CVB), 228
creativity, 16, 17, 61, 160, 224, 233, 245
  5th Chakra and, 114, 119
  personal chakra issue checklist, 65
Crohn's disease, *141,* 142, 265
crown chakra. *See* Chakra, 7th
curcumin, 127, 196, 212
cystitis, *160,* 168, 214–15

dairy, 66, 80, 131, 177, 198, 207, 231,
    237, 244, 252, 255, 259, 263,
    265
dancing, 170. *See also* pole dancing
dehydration, 223, 239, 243
dental care, 115, 131
depression, 205–8
  4th Chakra and, 130
  6th Chakra and, 94
  addiction and, 201–2
  chronic fatigue syndrome and, 223
  personal chakra issue checklist, 63
  treatment options, 206–8
Descartes, René, 92–93
detoxing, 64, 80, 95–97, 178, 190, 252
DHA, 196
DHEA, 260, 278
diabetes, *141,* 225–30
  low sugar and, 226–27
  risk factors of, 227–29
  treatment options, 229–30
diet, 80, 230–31
  3rd Chakra and, 143
  4th Chakra and, 131
  for acid reflux, 197–98
  for ADHD, 200
  for adrenal glands, 204
  for autoimmune diseases, 212
  for bone health, 219
  chronic dieting, 143, 145–49
  for depression, 207
  for diabetes, 229–30
  for gallbladder, 237–38
  for gut issues, 262–23
  for immune system, 244
  for Lyme disease, 252
  for PCOS, 255
  personal chakra issue checklist,
    64, 66
  plant-based (vegetarian), 131, 177,
    216, 230–31, 255
  for thyroid issues, 117–18
dissociation, 165
distractions, 44, 63
DMT (N-dimethyltryptamine), 93
dopamine, 141
dream interpretation, 50–51, 79, 109
drinking water, 143, 204, 223
  personal chakra issue checklist,
    64, 66

dry eyes, 268
dysfunctional families. *See* family dysfunction
dyslexia, 247

eating disorders, 145–55, 242. *See also* bulimia
  addressing issues about food and your body, 152–55
  chronic dieting, 145–49
  signs and symptoms of, 151
electronic frequency machines, 252
ELISA test, 249
EMDR (eye movement desensitization and reprocessing), 169–70, 202, 233
emotional cleansing, 98–103
emotional root causes. *See* root causes
emotional sensitivity, 55, 129, 132, 135–36, 199, 201
empaths, *75,* 55, 103, *130,* 133–36
  advice for, 134–35
  common traits of, 133
  personal chakra issue checklist, 63–64
endocarditis, 221–22
endometriosis, *160,* 168, 233
energy healing, 9, 10, 30, 204, 214, 253
  connecting to intuition through, 53
  resources, 275–76
"energy vampires," 99
EPA (eicosapentaenoic acid), 196
epigenetics, 119, 124, 179–80, 209
Epsom salt baths, 96, 102
Epstein-Barr virus (EBV), 224, 234, 249–50, 254, 265–67
estrogen, 65, 96, 218, 242, 278
evil, 40–42. *See also* negative energy and people
  6th Chakra and, 95, 98–101
exercise, 231–32
  3rd Chakra and, 143
  4th Chakra and, 131
  for ADHD, 200
  for adrenal glands, 204
  for bone health, 218
  chronic fatigue syndrome and, 223
  hormone imbalance and, 242
  for immune system, 244
  for PCOS, 255
  for sleep, 260
  weight and body image, 148
eyebright, 267

family dysfunction, 179–87
  5th Chakra and, 120–27
  7th Chakra and, 83, *83*
  author's story, 2, 16, 17, 24–25, 121–25, 181–82
  breaking the cycle, 185–87
  case study, Derek, 126–27
  case study, Sheila, 187–90
  common roles in, 182–83
  diabetes and, 226
  personal chakra issue checklist, 65
  sexual dysfunction and, 233
fasting, 21, 96, 150
fatigue, 126, 133, 203, 206, 236, 250. *See also* chronic fatigue syndrome
fears (fearfulness), 63, 88–89, 90–91
ferritin, 117, 177, 215–17, 248
fertility, *160,* 232–34
fibromyalgia, 234, 253–54
fight-or-flight response, 131, 203, 207, 227
flavonoids, 263
flaxseed, 210, 222
flu shots, 24, 121–22, 211–12
food allergies and intolerances, 235–37, 264
  6th Chakra and, 95
food diaries, 154, 236–37
forgiveness, 185

GABA, 141, 261
gallbladder, *141,* 142, 237–38
garlic, 210, 221–22, 229, 248
generational trauma. *See* family dysfunction
genetic predisposition, 179–80, 209, 211, 226
GERD (gastroesophageal reflux disease), 196–98
gestational diabetes, 228
ginkgo biloba, 261, 267
Global Lyme Alliance, 248, 249
glutathione, 212

gluten, *66*, 80, 131, 177, 207, 236, 244, 252, 255, 258, 265
gluten-free food brands, 278
God, 28–29, 41, 42–43, 64, 80, 82
goitrogens, 117–18
Graves's disease, *113*, 116–17, 212
green color, *49*, 129
Greenleaf, Linda, 103
green tea, 118, 210, 229, 248, 263
grief
    4th Chakra and, 130, *130*
    6th Chakra and, 104, 105
    7th Chakra and, 83
    personal chakra issue checklist, 63
    sexual abuse and, 168
Grof, Stanislav and Christina, 86–87
grounding, 56, 85, 102, 133, 245
    exercise, 103
guides, use of term, 28
Guillain-Barré syndrome, 142, 211–12
guilt, 63, 70, 126, 133, 149, 168
gut, 133, 219
    3rd Chakra and, *141*, 141–42, 143, 144
    immune system and, 142, 244
    personal chakra issue checklist, 63
    probiotics for healthy. *See* probiotics
    ulcers, *H. pylori* bacteria, and, 262–64
"gut feelings," 140, 144
gut imbalance, 155, 206, 246, 247

hand washing, 244
Hashimoto's thyroiditis, 60, 104, *113*, 114, 116, 212
Hay, Louise, 48, 57
headaches, 238–40
    6th Chakra and, *93*, 104–5
    acid reflux and, 197
    anxiety and depression, 206
    blood diseases and, 216
    fibromyalgia and, 234
    food allergies and, 236
    low blood sugar and, 227
    root causes of, 168, 238–40
    stress and, 60, 239
Healing Touch (HT), 253, 275
health insurance, 59, 60, 249
heartburn, 236
heart chakra. *See* Chakra, 4th

heart disease. *See* cardiovascular disease
heart palpitations, *126*, 135, 217, 235
    anxiety and depression, 205
heart rate, 131, 227
Helicobacter pylori (H. pylori), 262–63
helicopter parenting, 63, *130*, 136
hemochromatosis, 177, 248
hemorrhoids, 240–41
herxing, 241
high blood pressure (hypertension), 79, 126, 197, 215–16, 229, 243
histamine, 231, 257–58
hormone imbalances, 241–42
    2nd Chakra and, *160*
    anxiety and depression, 205
    chronic fatigue syndrome and, 224
    cystitis and, 215
    headaches and, 239
    sleep and, 259, 260
hormone replacement, 215, 218
hydration, 64, 66, 96, 143, 204, 223
hydration. *See* drinking water
"hygiene hypothesis," 235
hyperthyroidism, 113, 116
hypnotherapy (hypnosis), 210–11
hypoadrenalism, 203, 204
hypoglycemia, 225–30
hypophosphatemia, 197
hypothalamus, *93*, 117
hypothyroidism, 116
    personal chakra issue checklist, 66, *66*
hysterectomies, 17

"illnesses," 1
immune system, 243–45
    1st Chakra and, *176*
    3rd Chakra and, *141*, 141–42
    6th Chakra and, 96
    case study, Caroline, 137
    detoxing, 96
    "hygiene hypothesis" and, 235
    strengthening and protecting, 243–45
    stress and, 60
indigo color, 92
inflammation, 246
insulin resistance, 225–30
interstitial cystitis, *160*, 214–15

intimacy, 70, *130,* 160, *160,* 162, 167, 233, 256, 259
intuition, 7–8, 37
  6th Chakra and, 93–94
  connection to. *See* connecting to intuition
  defined, 37–38
  use of term, 28
Intuitive Soul Painting, 45–49, 77, 270
  author's sample, 29, 34–35, *35*
  creating your own, 47–48
  interpreting and symbolism, 48–49, *49*
Intuitive Writing Prompts
  1st Chakra, 177
  2nd Chakra, 161
  3rd Chakra, 143
  4th Chakra, 130–31
  5th Chakra, 114
  6th Chakra, 95
  7th Chakra, 83–84
  for Lyme disease, 250–51
iodine, 114, 117, 224
iron, 177, 216–17. *See also* ferritin
irritability, 40, 164, 197, 199, 200, 205, 216, 226
irritable bowel syndrome (IBS), 55, 126, 142, 212

journaling. *See* Intuitive Writing Prompts; Written Dialogue
Jung, Carl (Jungian psychology), 1, 3, 7, 13, 19, 21–23, 27, 37, 55, 59, 82, 92, 112, 129, 140, 159, 175
  dream interpretation, 50–51
  intuition and, 37–38
  The Red Book, 89–90
  the Shadow, 119

Kabat-Zinn, Jon, 102
ketogenic diet, 256
kidney stones, 237
knee problems, 246–47
Kundalini yoga, 88, 97, 276

L-carnitine, 213
learning disabilities, *93,* 247
L-glutamine, 212, 261
life purpose of author, 10, 19–26

listening to your intuition. *See* connecting to intuition
liver, *141,* 142, 226, 247–48
  3rd Chakra and, 143
love, 2, 3, 13, 27, 38, 41, 100, 102
low blood pressure, 203, 215–16, 243
Lucas, Catherine G., 86–87
lutein, 267
Lyme disease, 60, 248–53
  1st Chakra and, 187, 188–89
  anxiety and depression, 206, 208
  author's story, 14, 56–57, 208, 250
  headaches and, 239
  herxing and, 241
  learning disabilities and, 247
  resources, 274
  symptoms of, 206, 234, 239, 248–49
  testing for, 249
  treatment options, 250–53

magenta color, *49,* 188
magnesium, 204, 219, 229, 239, 278
malabsorption, 137, 155, 200, 212, 223, 232–33
Maladhara. See Chakra, 1st
Manipura. See Chakra, 3rd
medical intuition, 2–3, 25–26, 109
  author's story, 2, 8, 10, 16, 19, 22–26
medical intuitive reading of author, 10, 11, 14, 27–36
  intuitive painting, 29, 34–35, 35
  report, 29, *31–34*
  use of chakras, 29–30
  working with guides, 28–29
medical marijuana, 252
medications. *See also specific medications*
  personal chakra issue checklist, 65–66
meditation, 88, 102, 110, 200, 204, 260. *See also* mindfulness meditation
  connecting to intuition through, 53
mediumship classes, 24, 109
melatonin, 92–93, 260
menopause, 146, 215, 241–42, 260
menstrual problems, 239, 253, 264
mercury fillings, 115
metabolism, 21, 143, 147, 148, 223

migraine headaches, 238–40
  6th Chakra and, *93,* 104–5
  case study, Sheila, 188
  personal chakra issue checklist, *67*
milk-alkali syndrome, 197
mindfulness meditation, 44–45, 85,
  88, 102, 200, 211
mold
  4th Chakra and, 130
  6th Chakra and, *93,* 95, 98, 137, 172
  ADHD and, 200
  anxiety and depression, 206, 208
  asthma and, 209
  headaches and, 239
  Lyme disease and, 250, 251
  personal chakra issue checklist,
    64, 66
  resources, 274
  sinus issues and, 258
  thyroid dysfunction and, 117
mood swings, 199, 200–201
movement, 231–32. *See also* exercise
MTHFR (methylene tetrahydrofolate
  reductase), 223–24
multiple sclerosis (MS), 253–54, 266
myocarditis, 221–22
"mystical experience," 40

narcissism, 94, *141,* 179, 220
nature, immersion in, 102, 110, 245
nausea, 197, 217, 227, 264
neck alignment, *113,* 177
neck injuries, 261
negative energy and people, 98–103
  case study, "Amy," 104–6
  immune system and, 245
  as obstacle to connecting to
    intuition, 40–42
  sexual abuse and, 168–69
  ways to protect against, 89, 102–3
negative thinking, 13–14, *45,* 81, 97,
  164
neurological disorders, 253–54
nightmares, 50, 51, 164, 227
nitrates, 118, 196

occupational asthma, 209
omega-3 oils, 127, 196, 200, 210, 213,
  248, 267
oracle cards, 51–52

orange color, *49,* 159
orthorexia, 150–51
osteopathy, 210
osteopenia, 217
osteoporosis, 217–19
overthinking, 37, 39, 230, 239

painting. *See* Intuitive Soul Painting
panic attacks, *130,* 137, 167, 242
parasites, 206, 208, 251, 264
"patient-based root cause medicine,"
  60
pendulums, 52–53
peony, 213
perchlorates, 118
perfectionism, 141, 183, 202
pericarditis, 221–22
pesticides, 95–96, 118, 196
pineal gland, 83, 92–93
pituitary glands, *93,* 117
pole dancing, 66, 148, 218, 232
polycystic ovary syndrome (PCOS),
  168, 218, 228, 242, 254–56
postpartum depression, 242
poverty, 125, 179
pregnancy, 123–24, 242, 243
  author's story, 23–24
premenstrual syndrome (PMS), *160,*
  253
probiotics, 127, 143, 197, 208, 209,
  213, 244, 258, 262, 263, 278
psoriasis, 212, 221
psychic abilities, 39, 42, 64
  quiz about, 106–9
  tips for increasing, 109–10
psychometry, 109
PTSD (post-traumatic stress
  disorder), 162–67
  case study, Jill, 171–73
  healing strategies for, 169–71
  symptoms of, 164–66, 220

radiation treatments, 214, 218
Raynaud's disease, 224–25
rBGH (recombinant bovine growth
  hormone), 231
Red Book, The (Jung), 89–90
red color, *49,* 175, 215
red yeast rice, 222
Reiki, 97, 202, 214, 253, 275

rejection, fear of, 61, 113, 119, 133, 165, 220
Resch, Elyse, 146
resveratrol, 212, 222, 229
role models, 18, 114, 177
root causes, 3–4, 7–8, 9, 14–15, 59–61
  1st Chakra, 176, *176*
  2nd Chakra, 160, *160*
  3rd Chakra, *141,* 141–42
  4th Chakra, 130, *130*
  5th Chakra, *113,* 113–14
  6th Chakra, *93,* 94–95
  7th Chakra, 83, *83*
  personal chakra issue checklist, 62–67
root chakra. *See* Chakra, 1st
runes, 53

sacral chakra. *See* Chakra, 2nd
Sahasrara. See Chakra, 7th
saw palmetto, 242
schizophrenia, 90, 180, 266
scleroderma, 212, 221
scoliosis, 176, 214
seizures, *93,* 227, 240, 256–57
selenium, 114, 210
self-acceptance, 13, 78, 170
self-esteem, 29, 62, 95, 201–2
  3rd Chakra and, 140–41, *141*
  5th Chakra and, 113, 115, 119
self-love, 2, 13, 16, 21, 27, 78, 170, 201, 207, 222, 254
serotonin, 141, 230
sexual abuse or assault, 162–63, 167–71
  case study, Jill, 171–73
  emotional and physical effects of, 168
  healing strategies for, 169–71
  symptoms of, 167–68
sexual dysfunction, *160,* 168, 232–34
sexual identity, 160, 168–69
shame, 7, 16, 61, 121, 123–24, 144, 146, 149, 151, 155, 159, 160, 168
shoulder injuries, 261
shoulder pain, 115
sinus issues, 219, 236, 239, 257–58
Sjögren's syndrome, 105, 238
skin conditions, 258–59
  1st Chakra and, 176, *176,* 177

autoimmune diseases and, 212
case study, "Amy," 104
case study, Caroline, 136
sleep
  for ADHD, 200
  for adrenal glands, 204
  for diabetes, 229
  for gut health, 263
  for immune system, 244
sleep habits, 259–61
sleep issues
  anxiety and, 205
  chronic fatigue syndrome and, 223
  headaches and, 239
  inflammation and, 246
  nightmares, 50, 51, 164, 227
  as obstacle to connecting with intuition, 40
  personal chakra issue checklist, 65
  PTSD and, 164
smoking, 115, 118, 131, 196, 209, 218, 221, 225, 243, 263
solar plexus chakra. *See* Chakra, 3rd
Soul Painting. *See* Intuitive Soul Painting
soy foods, 118, 242
speleotherapy, 211
spiritual awakening, 83–89
spiritual crisis, 83, *83,* 85–89
  The Red Book and Jung's, 89–90
spiritual guides of author, 28–29
Spiritualist churches, 24, 109
spiritual root causes. *See* root causes
spironolactone, 256
steroids, 219, 244, 259
stiff neck and shoulders, 261
stomach ulcers, 262–64
stress, 60–61
  2nd Chakra, 161
  5th Chakra and, 114
  chronic fatigue syndrome and, 223
  depression and, 206
  fertility and sexual dysfunction issues, 233–34
  gut health and, 263
  headaches and, 60, 239
  personal chakra issue checklist, 64
stress relief, 170–71
  for immune system, 244
  for sleep, 260

substance abuse. *See* addiction
sunglasses, 268
supplements, 195–96. *See also specific*
supplements
  for autoimmune diseases, 212–13
  labels, 196
  for Lyme disease, 252
  personal chakra issue checklist,
    63, 65–66
  for sleep, 260
support network, 64, 66
Sutherland, Jean, 20, 21–22, 38
Svadhisthana. See Chakra, 2nd
symptoms, 10, 55–58

teeth, and 5th Chakra, 57, *113*
teeth care, 115, 131
teeth grinding, *113,* 116, 239
testosterone, 65, 218, 242, 256, 259
third eye chakra. *See* Chakra, 6th
throat chakra. *See* Chakra, 5th
thyroid, 60, 104, *113,* 114, 115, 116–20
  expressing your feelings to
    support, 119–20
thyroid stimulating hormone (TSH)
  tests, 116–17
tinnitus, 261–62
tonsillitis, *68, 113*
toxins. *See also* mold
  3rd Chakra and, 142
  6th Chakra and, *93,* 95–96
  anxiety and depression, 207
  asthma and, 209
  detoxing, 64, 80, 95–97, 178, 190, 252
  inflammation and, 246
  Lyme disease and, 252
traditional Chinese medicine (TCM),
  57, 226, 238, 239, 248, 254
trance states, 21, 89–90
transgender, 169
trauma, 11, 13–14, 15–18. *See also*
  PTSD
  5th Chakra and, 113
  6th Chakra and, 94
  7th Chakra, 83, *83*
  as obstacle to connecting with
    intuition, 40
Tribole, Evelyn, 146
tryptophan, 230
turkey, 230

twelve-step programs, 87, 143, 157,
  182, 202
Tylenol, 143, 248

ulcers, 262–64

vaccines, 121–25, 178, 211–12
vagus nerve, 141–42, 256
valerian root, 207, 260
van der Kolk, Bessel, 15, 165
varicose veins, *176,* 177
vegetarian (plant-based) diet, 131,
  177, 216, 230–31, 255
violet color, 82
viruses, 265–67. *See also specific*
  viruses
Vishuddha. See Chakra, 5th
vision problems, 267–68
  blurred/impaired vision, 104, 227
visualizations
  1st Chakra, 178
  2nd Chakra, 162
  3rd Chakra, 144
  4th Chakra, 132
  5th Chakra, 116
  6th Chakra, 98
  7th Chakra, 85
vitamin A, 267
vitamin C, 204, 216, 267
vitamin D, 213, 219
vitamin K, 219, 222
vitiligo, 212
vulnerability, 56, 90, 115, 121, 160, 233

water filtration, 64, 96
weight gain, 20–21, 56, 60, 131,
  146–47
weight issues, 145–49
weight loss, 147–48
weight scale, 148, 154
weight scales, 148, 154
white noise, 260
worrying, 44, 48, 55, 78, 98, 116, 130
Written Dialogue, 42–45, 88. *See also*
  Intuitive Writing Prompts

yellow color, *49,* 140
yoga, 53, 88, 97, 210, 276

zinc, 114, 210, 263, 267

CHAKRA CHART WORKSHEET			
Emotional		Physical	
7TH CHAKRA		**7TH CHAKRA**	
(Crown) Purpose in life, relationship with spirit		Life-threatening illnesses, chronic illnesses, brain, nervous system, overview of the body and spirit	
6TH CHAKRA		**6TH CHAKRA**	
(Third eye) Intuition, psychic ability, ability to perceive and make judgments about the world, morality, flexibility, ability to change and fit into society without changing so much that you lose yourself, mood, mental illness		Headaches, including migraines; vision and hearing issues; sensitivity to mold, chemicals, scents, and other toxins; brain tumor; stroke; neurological diseases or injury	
5TH CHAKRA		**5TH CHAKRA**	
(Throat) Self-expression—too much or not enough, will and determination, making things happen vs. waiting for things to happen, communication authenticity, activism, judgment, and criticism		Thyroid issues, dental problems, teeth grinding, acid reflux, neck alignment or injury, rotator-cuff injuries, tonsillitis, chronic sore throat	
4TH CHAKRA		**4TH CHAKRA**	
(Heart) Expressing emotions—too much or not enough, love, intimacy, nurturing, grief, parenting—helicopter or neglect, giving vs. getting help, being an empath, sensitivity, self vs. others—boundaries, codependency		Heart disease, blood pressure, cancer of any of these areas, asthma, COPD, lungs, breasts, pneumonia, bronchitis	

Emotional		Physical	
3RD CHAKRA		**3RD CHAKRA**	
(Solar plexus) Eating disorders, body image, self-esteem—not enough or narcissism, responsibility to yourself vs. others, self-care, perfectionism, ability to take criticism, pride		Gut and bowel issues, bacterial imbalance, food intolerances, ulcers, liver disease, addiction, adrenals, weight concerns, diabetes	
2ND CHAKRA		**2ND CHAKRA**	
(Sacral) Feminine/masculine energy balance, abuse trauma, creativity, career and work vs. personal time, intimacy, sexuality, including sexual identity		Fertility, PMS, endometriosis, fibroids, polycystic ovary syndrome, urinary problems, hormone imbalance, menopause, sexual dysfunction, back pain	
1ST CHAKRA		**1ST CHAKRA**	
(Root) Family issues and family history, trust, safety, basic needs, caretaking, support systems and belonging, healthy boundaries		Blood diseases; autoimmune disorders; immune deficiency; AIDS; bones, joints, and muscles; skin; general inflammation; varicose veins; sciatica	

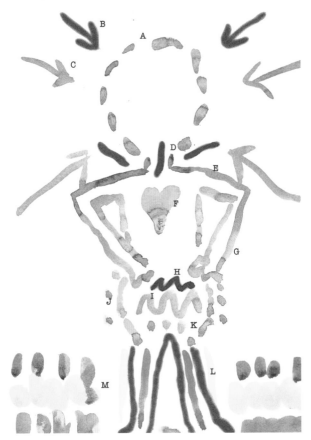

PAINTING THREE

A. Red in the head (the 7th chakra) symbolizes anxiety for this person regarding health concerns and the future but the dotted lines indicate openness to spirit.

B. Spirit sending in healing energy and positivity.

C. Blue arrows indicate this person is sensitive, empathic, and picking up energy from others around them. This energy may be invasive and they may have trouble setting boundaries.

D. The 5th chakra is about expression and this person struggles with that. The purple indicates that anxiety is not necessary and that they need to listen to their intuition to guide them. The lines extending out mean that expressing themselves will create more intuitive connections.

E. The wide shoulders mean stress, "the weight of the world on their shoulders." In this case blue is an indication that they feel that they need to take care of the many people who depend on them.

F. A red heart is a sign of passion as well as anger for this person.

G. The hands on the hips is a sign of defiance, symbolically expressing that this person has had enough of being underappreciated.

H. A signal to listen to their intuition and gut feelings.

I. Blue in the gut often means that the person is picking up their own and other people's feelings here. Gut-related symptoms are signals to tune into their feelings, then ask if they belong to them or if they are picking the feelings up from someone else.

J. Red in the gut often is a sign of trauma related to the 2nd chakra, such as sexual abuse or assault. It can also be a sign of a medical issue or pain here such as miscarriage, hip pain, or disorders related to the reproductive organs. The fact that not only is the hip area red but also that red dots surround the area means that both trauma and health issues are present.

K. Red dots in the 1st chakra signal that the person's childhood and early life were difficult.

L. This person is moving forward as an intuitive, generous, spiritual teacher (yellow), fueled by spirit (purple) and courage (orange).

M. Grounding and being present will help bring about courage, inspiration to be a spiritual teacher, and growth and new life (green).